Hair
POWER

TO MY CHILDREN, HARRISON AND TELLISA

Hair
POWER

Nicky Clarke

with Jo Foley

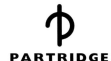

PARTRIDGE

LONDON · NEW YORK · TORONTO · SYDNEY · AUCKLAND

TRANSWORLD PUBLISHERS LTD, 61—63 Uxbridge Road, London W5 5SA

TRANSWORLD PUBLISHERS (AUSTRALIA) PTY LTD, 15—25 Helles Avenue, Moorebank, NSW 2170

TRANSWORLD PUBLISHERS (NZ) LTD, 3 William Pickering Drive, Albany, Auckland

Published 1999 by Partridge a division of Transworld Publishers Ltd

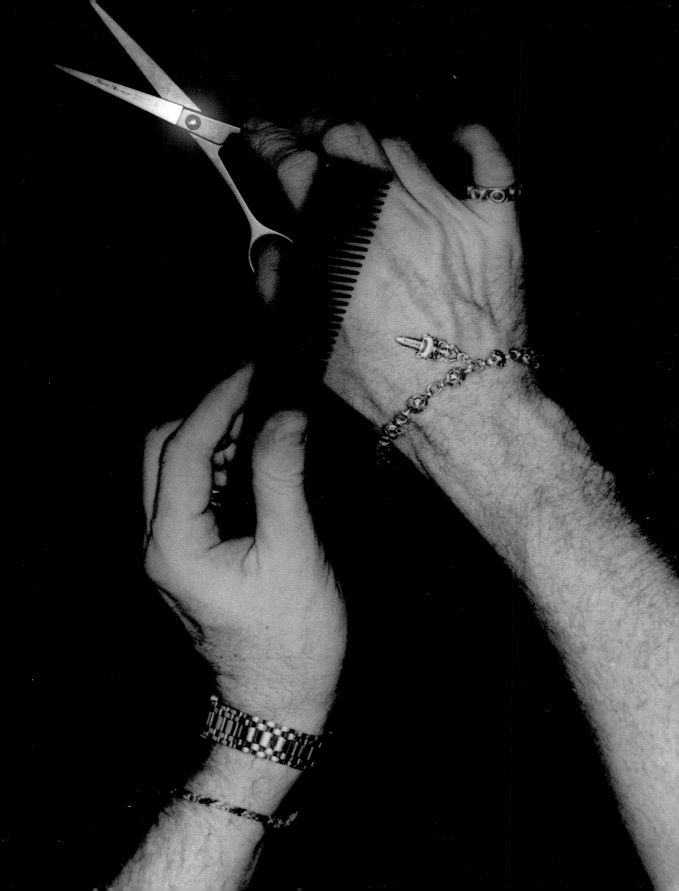

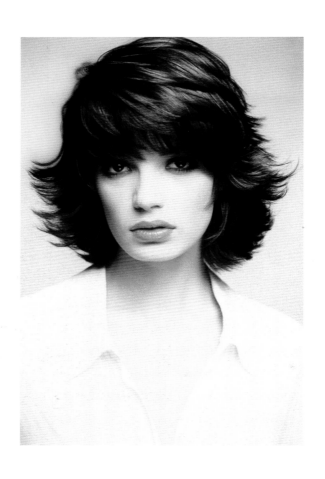

'I know that if you can help somebody *look* better, they will immediately *feel* better, and that a new hairstyle or cut is one of the best ways to do this. It doesn't have to be a drastic change. Indeed, sometimes it's better if it isn't. I want to add a little something, not force a new personality on someone.'

Nicky Clarke

contents

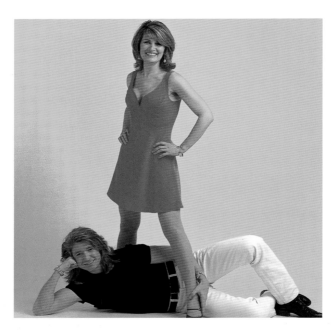

Writing this book gives me the opportunity to acknowledge the many people who have helped to make my journey possible. There have, of course, been many. One person, however, stands head and shoulders (if you'll pardon the pun) above anyone else: my wife and business partner, Lesley Clarke (Managing Director of Nicky Clarke worldwide).

Without Lesley my journey would not have begun, let alone succeeded beyond my wildest dreams. It was Lesley's idea to open our own prestige Mayfair salon – complete with a celebrity and royal clientele. It was her faith in my ability that led us to break the much-publicized £100 haircut barrier, and we've never looked back.

Together we launched the Nicky Clarke signature hair care products – Hairomatherapy (inspired by Lesley's passion for aromatherapy), Sport and Men. Lesley's sound business acumen, drive and strong marketing savvy, combined with her push to promote me personally in the media, have led to massive public awareness.

She is also the mother of my two wonderful children. My debt to her is immense, and I am really pleased to be able to acknowledge it here.

Introduction

Hair is powerful. Touchable, seductive, sexy and strong. It is truly amazing stuff. My work has taken me on an incredible adventure into a dazzling world of glamour and excitement. I'm thrilled to be able to share that with you here.

This very personal book charts some of my experiences from my early days in hairdressing as a junior stylist at Leonard of Mayfair — at the time the most exclusive and glamorous salon in London — to my travels around the world many times over as one of the most sought-after photo-session hair stylists in the business. Then onwards to my current busy media-based lifestyle, and the huge success of my signature hair care product ranges. It's been quite a journey!

In *Hair Power* I trace the history of hair care and style in the twentieth century, and examine the areas and hair care problems that most concern my own clients and my TV audiences and — I'm sure — women and men the length and breadth of the country. In *Hair Power* you'll find sections on confidence, the art of looking seductive, feeling good and looking good, transforming your hair image, colouring, perming, choosing the right style for you, long hair, short hair, hair care, problem solving — and much more!

Hair has never been such a hot media subject — just look at all the magazines and TV stories that appear on a daily basis — and it seems that the demand for hair knowledge is insatiable. We are all in the process of rediscovering and enjoying hair as the ultimate fashion accessory — and we want to know more. I hope that this book will inspire, and convey my passion for Hair Power.

NICKY CLARKE

snip...

The rain was unreal – it came down in floods, like a backwash gone mad. In seconds everyone was soaked and the sheet of rain was so dense you could hardly see the stage. Umbrellas were going up and somebody was doing a roaring trade in black bin-liners. I was sitting at home watching the whole thing on TV, my head in my hands, not believing what I was seeing.

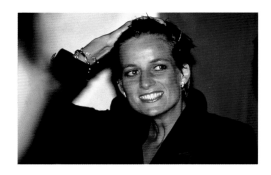

Princess Diana looked stunning – eyes shining, head thrown back laughing. Pity about her hair, though. The downpour on the night of the open-air Pavarotti concert in Hyde Park ensured my handiwork was never really appreciated by the crowds.

Earlier in the day I'd had a call from one of my clients, the Duchess of York. Could I come to the Palace and do her hair for an event that evening, she asked. We'd already pencilled something in the diary, so I knew I might be needed. All we had to do was agree a convenient time. Just before she put the phone down, she asked if I could possibly do the hair of a friend who might be with her when I arrived. What do you say under the circumstances but yes?

So here I was, waiting to see the friend, whose hair I'd just done for the first time, on the TV in the downpour. Eventually the rain began to clear and the conductor and orchestra reassembled. The crowd went quiet and then a very large man walked on stage to tumultuous applause, bowed and blew a kiss to somebody in the front row. The cameras panned and there, smiling back at Pavarotti, with her hair soaking wet and plastered to her head, was the Princess of Wales. So much for my handiwork!

snip...

I walked past the door a couple of times before I realized it was the right address. A huge, elegant house on the corner of Grosvenor Square. In my hurry I hadn't seen the discreet brass plaque outside. I walked past again before I realized this was the door I was looking for. As I went in I knew that this was what I wanted. There were chandeliers and antiques, a large curving staircase with wrought-iron banisters and a hum that said more about style and money than I'd ever dreamed of. I felt a bit like Alice going through the looking glass, wide-eyed and open-mouthed and desperately trying to look as cool and sophisticated as a sixteen-year-old south London boy could in the heart of Mayfair. I decided at that moment that this was where I belonged. I'd just been offered a job at a prestigious Sloane Street salon, but *this* was where I wanted to be. I'd arrived at Leonard's for my interview. The most beautiful and most creative salon in the capital. An hour later all they said was that they would let me know.

snip...

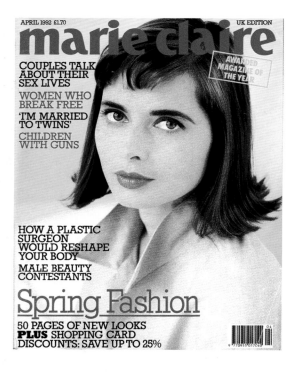

The face in the mirror looking at me was one I'd seen hundreds of times blown up on a large screen. It was probably one of the most beautiful ever made. Huge blue eyes, cheekbones so high they could give Everest a run for its money and a mouth full and wide. As a kid I'd seen that face in old black-and-white movies. It had held generations captive. Yet here it was, living, breathing and looking much younger than I remembered. A quick pinch brought me back down to earth. The ravishing face in front of me belonged to Isabella Rossellini and I'd been asked to spend three days working with her. And to think I'd considered turning down the job because I hadn't wanted to spend that amount of time at a photographic session!

snip...

I was aware of her coming up the stairs but was busy finishing something else and didn't take much notice. Every so often I'd glance across to where she was sitting to see how things were. She seemed to be sinking lower and lower in her chair. Once or twice I caught sight of her in a mirror and she looked seriously nervous. I went over briefly to say hello and to look at her and her hair – she hardly said a word. When I eventually got to her she shook her head, listlessly saying that as she'd been waiting for five months for this appointment what did another hour matter. I explained that sometimes the new-client waiting list was long but hoped she would think the wait worthwhile. While I looked at her hair, examining the way it grew and noting its condition, I asked her if she had any ideas of how she wanted to wear it. She just smiled and told me to do whatever I liked.

This often happens – people come to me when they've tried everything else and are desperate. She was fed up with the way she looked and the way she felt about herself. She'd waited five months for an appointment, had caught a train from Leeds that morning and was about to part with £300 so that a man she had only read about could cut her hair. Some time later I watched her leave the salon. She held her head up – and her shoulders – and she even laughed as she handed over the money. Of course she looked better than when she'd come in, but she also felt much better about herself. That's the power of hair.

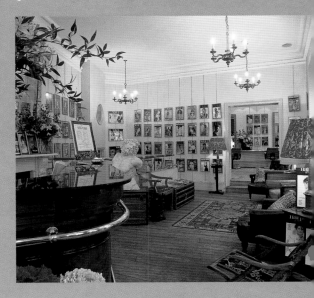

snip...

Someone recently asked me, hypothetically, whether I'd like to do the Queen's hair. Immediately I said yes, of course I would, I'd give anything to get my hands on it, I could make it look great – softer, prettier. And yet a part of me said no. There's something wonderful about that sort of Englishness, that belief that how you look is quite important but not *that* important. I admire the way she looks, so why should I change it?

In a way, that's why I've stayed on the shop floor all my working life. It's fun and glamorous to do photographic sessions and create wonderful looks and pictures, but it's not real. I've always felt the need to take some of the truly inspirational things we've done in the studio and see how they'd work in real life. That's why I continue to work in the salon with ordinary men and women and why I have only one salon instead of a string of them.

snip...

Backstage at fashion shows is manic and mind-blowing. It's also great fun and I love doing them. When I first started doing shows Anthony Price's were always the sharpest and most celebrity-filled because he made clothes for everybody from Bryan Ferry and Jerry Hall to Anjelica Huston. They were also the sexiest clothes you could imagine, and that's why he always got the best models around. It was wild working with them. One year I did a whole series of wigs which looked fantastic, particularly on the likes of Naomi Campbell and Yasmin Le Bon. It was a sort of chunky, slightly bitty, short bob. The girls all loved the style – but it was the guys watching the show who wanted the haircuts. Afterwards one of them came backstage to see his girlfriend and asked if I would do his hair like that. It was Nick Rhodes, and that's how I met Duran Duran and began to do their hair.

snip...

I'll always remember the phone call.

I'd been hanging around the house for nearly two weeks, even though I knew it would have been better to keep out of my dad's way. To say I was not in his good books is an understatement. My GCE results had been disastrous. Worse than any of my brothers' or sisters'. I'd taken refuge at my eldest sister's house and spent most of my time there. I even slept there. But somehow, after that interview, I had to be near home just in case they called. And they did. Two long weeks later, two of the longest weeks of my life, they called and offered me a junior's job at Leonard's. I was on my way.

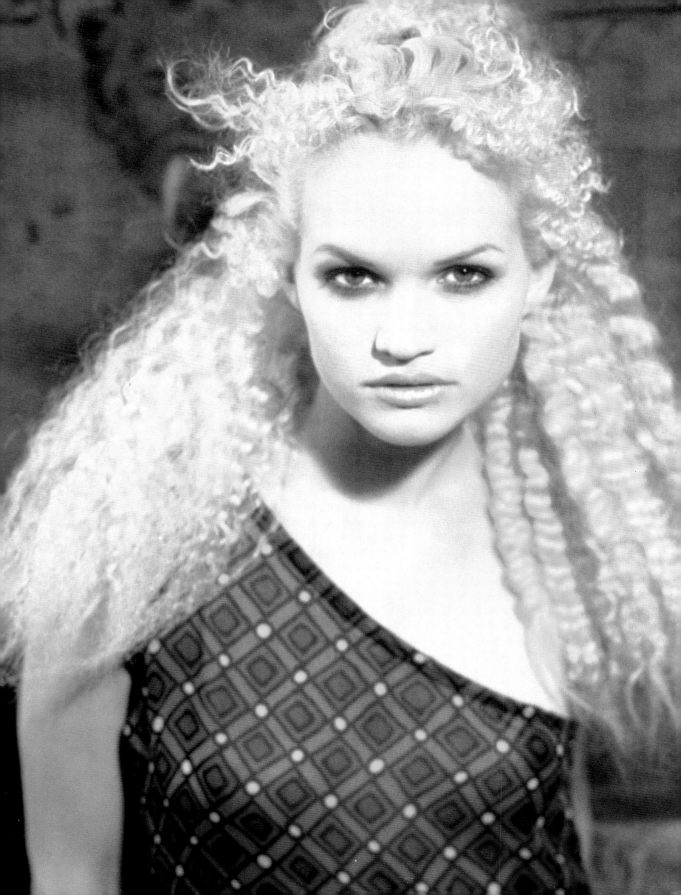

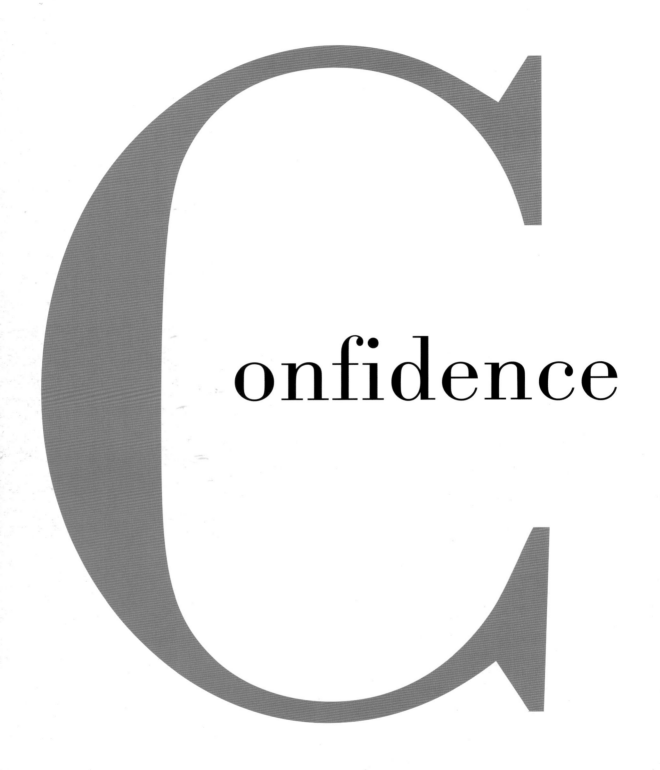

Confidence

Very few people have complete confidence in themselves – in what they do, how they look and who they are. We all need help from time to time. I know that better than most. Every week women come into my salon who lack confidence – I can tell by the way they walk. I also see women behind the scenes at *This Morning*, my regular TV slot, hoping that my makeover today will help change their lives.

But I also know that if you can help somebody *look* better, they will immediately *feel* better, and that a new hairstyle or cut is one of the best ways to do this. It doesn't have to be a drastic change. Indeed, it's better if it isn't. I want to add a little something, not force a new personality on someone.

Your hair is vital to your self-esteem. Ask any woman what is the single most important factor in feeling good about herself and she will invariably say her hair. If her hair is right, she feels fine. If she's having a bad time with her hair, no amount of primping and prettifying and no amount of expensive designer clothes will make her feel better. Hence the expression Bad Hair Day!

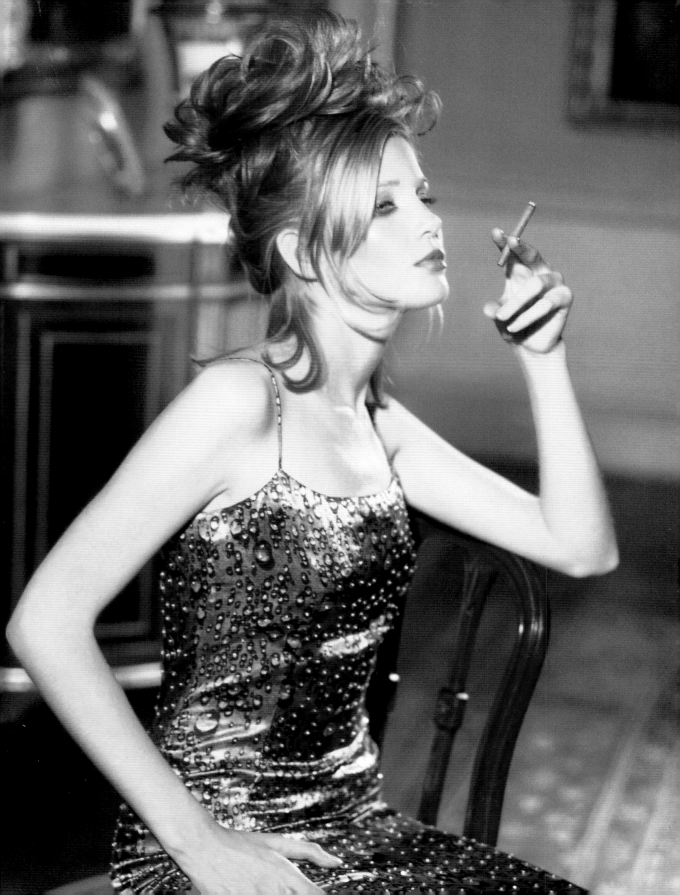

How you wear your hair makes a statement about who you are and what you are. You can strip everything away to a basic look: jeans, a white T-shirt and very little make-up, but your hair will still identify you. It's what makes the difference. It shows the world how you want to appear: well-groomed, wild, sporty, sexy, sophisticated, spontaneous, serious. Out of all the hundreds of thousands of hairstyles in the world, you chose a particular style and colour, and that says lots about you.

Most people believe that models, with their perfect figures, skin and hair, are super-confident, but even the most beautiful need help and

reassurance. I've worked with some of the world's top models and photographers

over the last twenty years, so I know what it takes to look that perfect – an army of

assistants, a make-up artist and a hairdresser constantly striving for perfection:

blotting a shiny nose here, trimming a wisp of hair there, hiding a spot, pinning a

curl. Add to that some great lighting and one of the world's top photographers and

of course you're going to get a great picture of a beautiful girl. And it can take a

whole day! With that sort of attention anyone could look terrific.

I started doing photographic sessions almost from the very beginning. I'd been at Leonard's only a couple of months when one of the top session stylists in town began to take me with him to sessions. My first was for *Vogue*. I could hardly believe what was happening – just turned sixteen and here I was nervously helping to get the models ready for a shoot with Barry Lategan – one of *the* great photographers of the Seventies. I remember everything about it. The models came into the salon for us to see their hair and discuss what could be done – it was a beautiful shoot, very elegant and grown-up. All the girls wore draped, Greek-goddess-style dresses, so the hair had to be kept simple. We just had to keep the lines clean and sharp. Because I'd made most of the hairpieces, I did the second day of the shoot on my own. And not long after that I did my first shoot on my own – with Lothar Schmidt, another of *Vogue*'s regular photographers. I could not believe my luck! Running about Mayfair, spending days at photographic studios, chatting up models …

I worked a lot with Sue Purdey, who was Barry Lategan's girlfriend at the time. I had the most amazing crush on her. I began to do her hair away from sessions too. She was such a successful model that she was always getting bookings and she would recommend me for the shoots. One of her best-known looks was Egyptian-inspired, and very inspirational. It was easy for me to do because I knew her hair well. I used to do it in the salon. The type of hair that looks great just washed and dried is very rare: most of us need more help, and that's what I tell my clients.

The studio work taught me a lot about how women like to look. Although I had a specific job to do at the studio, I always wanted the models to feel good about their hair when the session was over. I wanted them to like what I'd done. I also came to realize that what I was learning from the sessions I wanted to put into practice on people in real life. It was all very well doing perfect hair for the stillness of a magazine page, but I wanted to see it on someone walking down the street too.

But people, women in particular, can be hard on themselves. They have high expectations of how they should look, and this has intensified over the last ten years or so. They feel they should emulate what they see on TV and in the movies. All through the *Dallas* and *Dynasty* years many women felt they should be as well groomed and beautifully made-up as the lead players. What they may not have known about was the army of hair and make-up people it took even to make someone look dishevelled and sexy first thing in the morning. *Nobody wakes up looking like that!* Not real people, anyway.

People in the public eye are judged. The Duchess of York came in for a pounding, and that was undeserved. She was always compared with the Princess of Wales, which was unfair and unkind. People always said that Princess Diana looked fantastic, and she did. But she had a hairdresser in attendance every day. There'd be a photograph in the press of the Duchess of York taking her daughters to school or rushing to an appointment in the same paper as a glorious picture of the Princess of Wales, and the paper would say unkind things about how the duchess looked. That did terrible things to her confidence. What people failed to realize was that she only ever had her hair done when she was going out on an official function.

I started doing her hair before Princess Eugenie was born. I got a call one day from my good friend Terry O'Neill, one of the great photographers. He's been taking amazing pictures since the Sixties and has photographed many of the world's most beautiful women. He was doing a photo session, and suggested that I did the hair. I could hardly believe it when he told me that the subject was the Duchess of York, and that she'd okayed his choice of me.

The first time I drove up to the front gates of Buckingham Palace it was a scary experience. The police signalled me through the gates and I parked in full view of all the tourists. I was whisked through the Privy Purse entrance and taken upstairs by a footman. Eventually I arrived at the Duchess of York's private apartment and was ushered in.

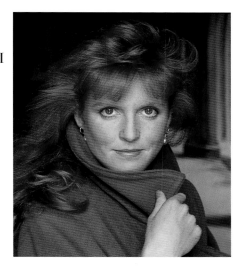

We got on fantastically well right from the beginning. She has great hair: it's very fine but there's an awful lot of it and it's very curly. It's a magical colour and in really good condition. She got to trust me and my judgement and I started doing her hair regularly.

Most of us keep our hair within the narrow parameters of a style and shape. It's probably one that suits us and that we've learnt how to manage. Every so often, however, we feel the urge to do something quite, quite different.

A woman is most likely to decide to do something radical with her hair when there has been a change in her life. And usually this is the end of a relationship. Then a woman will often ask for a shorter hairstyle – metaphorically she's giving the guy the chop and cutting him right out of her life.

I see this in the salon. A client arrives and blurts out that she would like something completely different. Although it's often the end of a relationship that brings a desire for a transformation – who'd want a sweeping change made in the looks that helped attract a current partner in the first place? – it isn't always. Mia Farrow dramatically changed her hair when she married Frank Sinatra. A lot of comment had been made about the difference in their ages and perhaps it got to Mia, who at that time had very long, pale blonde hair. She was so slender that it made her look waif-like. And instead of going for sophistication with chignons and pleats, which would have been inappropriate for her style, she decided to go for the chop and have an elfin cut. It made her look even younger and more vulnerable – but it gave her much more confidence and was a style she kept for years.

The Right Shape, the Right

There isn't one look for each individual. How dull life would be if there were – no fun, no drama and no experiments. It's the experiments, even when they don't work, that eventually create new looks and movements. And we all change throughout our lives. We change our cars, our wardrobes, our homes, our habits, our minds – so why not our hairstyles? Even those who appear to have had the same hairstyle all their lives almost certainly haven't. Take Jerry Hall, for instance – to most of us she seems always to have had that flowing 'southern belle' style. But she's been a client and so I know that she has had shorter hair, blonder hair, and has even had a fringe cut. Goldie Hawn is another: it may seem like the same look but in fact her hair has been long, short, straight, flicked up, curly, fringed and fringeless. Everybody needs a change occasionally. And we also need the mistakes because that's how we learn. I never tire of saying it – when you make a mistake with your hair, or think you have, it can always be rectified. *Hair is magic* – we can cut it, curl it, straighten it, colour it, shave it off, mistreat it, and it always comes back for more. Such loyalty deserves tender loving care – of which more later!

Most people like guidelines – if they know what the rules are they also know how far they can stretch or break them. One major consideration, when choosing a hairstyle, is your face shape. A good cut and a good technique can flatter the good points and disguise the weaker ones, for example by adding shape and shadow to a round face to help slim it down. So, on the following pages you'll find some rules. Just remember that they are not hard and fast.

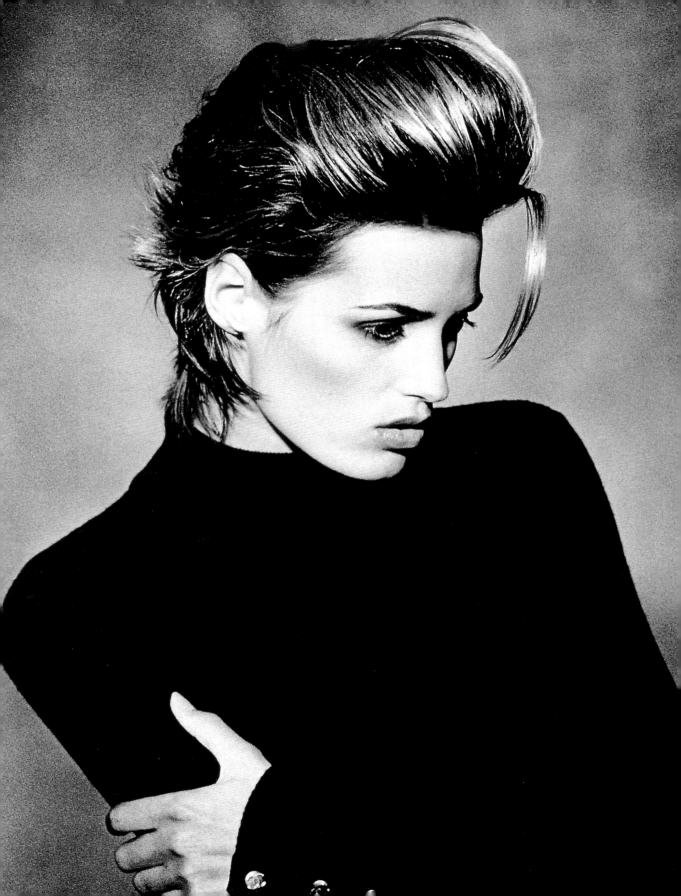

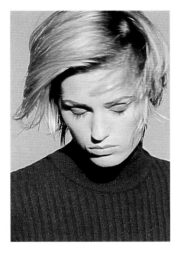 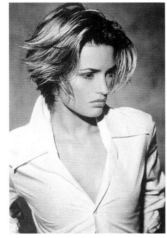 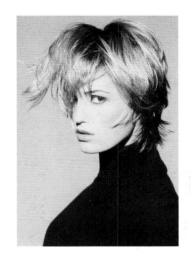

One of the most amazing photo sessions I ever worked on was with the supermodel Yasmin Le Bon. From a shoot lasting only two hours we got dozens of great pictures.

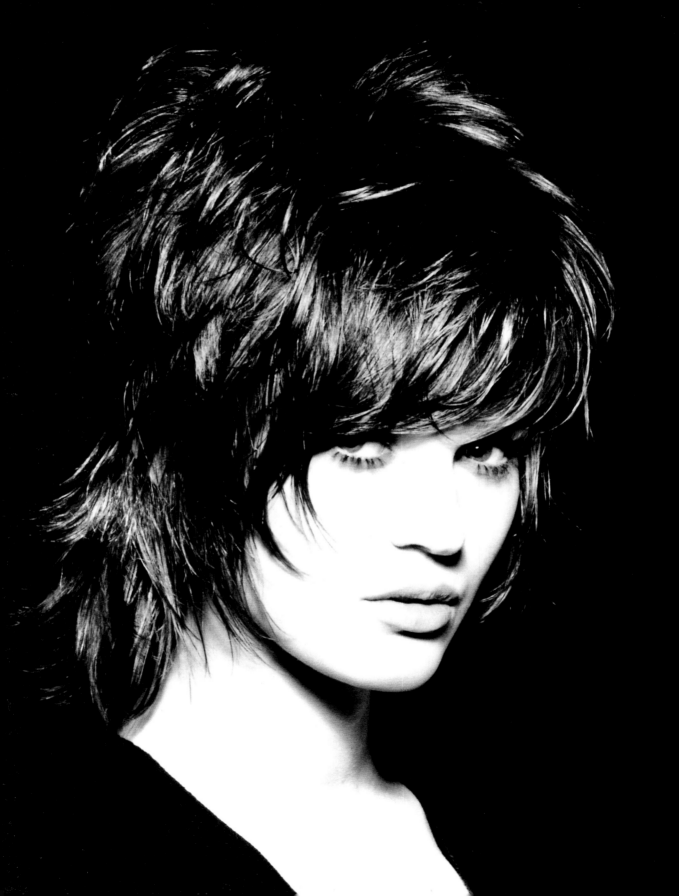

5 Face Shape

SQUARE Soft, wavy styles help soften sharp angles and harsh jawlines. Nothing too cropped or severe – no geometric cuts, scraped-back styles, heavy fringes or centre partings.

ROUND Soft cuts, graduated bobs, feathered styles and feathery fringes all add length and help slim the face. Avoid heavy fringes and curly styles, which only emphasize the roundness.

OVAL The perfect face shape – it can take any style, any length. Indeed, the idea of all other styles is to recreate that oval in square faces, round faces, long faces, and so on.

LONG The quickest, easiest and best way of minimizing the length is with a fringe. A curly bob or a style with width at the jaw also helps take the eye away from the length of the face. Avoid styles that lie flat at the side – they accentuate length.

HEART-SHAPED Balance the width of the top half of your face with styles that are fuller at the bottom, or have a bit of a kick or a flick-up.

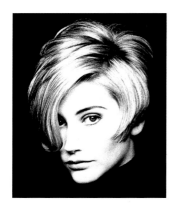

PROPORTIONS To work well, everything must be in proportion. When your hair is wet it'll show the shape of your head. Take a good long look at it. Does it need a style to add fullness at the sides or crown, or does it need more height and less width? Talk these things over with your hairdresser.

It is logical for a hairdresser to get on eye level with you. A hairdresser who's standing over a seated client cannot create a style for her – the proportions are all wrong. When people first saw me rolling across the salon in my chair they thought it was an affectation, but I've got to see how the hair looks and moves at the same level as the person it belongs to. I also believe that a hairdresser should always see you on your feet. I often get a client to stand up – even halfway through a restyle – just to check that my sense of her proportion is right.

How to find the style that gives you confidence

Make a list of the things you like best about yourself – everything from a sense of humour to your great legs or the fact that you're good with animals or kind to old ladies. Be honest, and generous – it's really important that you should recognize your good points.

Now write down everything you like about your hair and everything nice that anybody has ever said about it.

Now list what you don't like about it: it could be the colour, the way it frizzes up when you're exercising, or that you need to wash it every day and hate the tyranny of it.

Think of the last time you were happy with your hair and try to remember why: was it its length, its colour, its shape? Was it also that you were on holiday, or in love, or healthy and felt fit? Was it the shampoo you were using? Think of all the factors that contribute to feeling good about your hair as well as about yourself.

Collect pictures of styles you like. These will give your hairdresser an idea of what you're after, and he'll soon be able to tell you whether that style is right for your hair.

Be realistic. The style that will give you confidence is the one that suits your type of hair. If you have fine, flyaway hair it's best not to go for a pre-Raphaelite look. And a style that suits your hair will be one that you can manage too.

Now talk to your hairdresser. Discuss the matter thoroughly.

Be patient. You might not get the style of your dreams first or second time round. Both you and your hairdresser have to work with your hair – its length may not be quite right at first, or you might want to change the colour.

Be brave. Tell your hairdresser if you don't like it or it's not working. That way something can be done about it.

Admit it if you've made a mistake. Remember that you can always do something to rescue a hairstyle.

The Great Day

If there's one day in a woman's life when she needs all the confidence she can muster, it's her wedding day. She's probably fantasized about it since she was a little girl. It's the day when she's at the centre of the universe with everybody's attention on her. She's dreamt about it and planned it and she wants everything to be perfect. I've done the bride's hair for hundreds of weddings over the years and the most enjoyable occasions are always those where everything has been thoroughly planned and discussed.

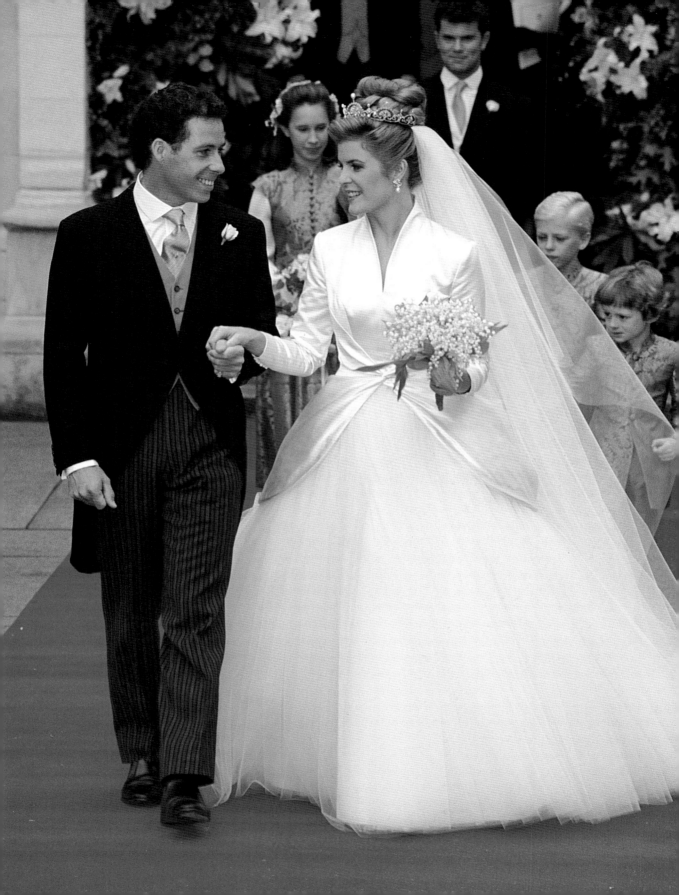

When Madeleine Gurdon married Andrew Lloyd Webber she wanted a traditional bridal look. We began to discuss her needs very early on in the planning process. For me, traditional doesn't mean dull. I do it with a twist, a little extra kick that redefines the tradition. Madeleine has good thick hair and it was relatively easy to design something around her headdress and veil, but we needed a couple of practice sessions so that everything felt right and she had nothing to worry about on the day.

It's amazing the number of things you have to think about – not just the dress and headdress but the length of the veil. Could it get caught by anything, by small bridesmaids or against old church pews? I thought I'd considered the lot over the years I'd been getting brides ready for their big day until I came to Serena Stanhope's wedding to Viscount Linley.

This is a wonderfully relaxed picture. I was thrilled to be asked to work on the engagement announcement shots for Viscount Linley and Serena Stanhope. The photographs broke new ground for 'official' royal portraits. The dress that the future Viscountess Linley wore was one that I borrowed from Lesley.

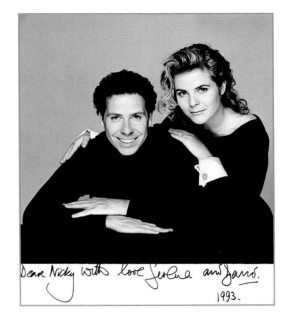

Serena had decided very early on that she wanted an elegant and classic look. She greatly admired the way her mother-in-law, Princess Margaret, had looked on her wedding day, and she wanted a similar polish to her look. On the day she looked glorious – she had a classic Grace Kelly elegance. Her hairstyle was intricate at the back with lots of knotting and plaiting, and very smooth and sleek at the front. She has what I call English-type hair – not too fine, not too thick – which is very good to work with because it can be either sleek or wavy. I was invited to Kensington Palace on a number of occasions before the wedding and I helped her choose her tiara. We had practice runs with the tiara, and more practice runs with the tiara and veil. But what none of us had taken into account in all the excitement was the height of her hairstyle. It looked wonderfully graceful but on the big day it bashed against the roof of the car as she arrived at Westminster Abbey. That's why there were photographs in all the papers of me rushing to the rescue to straighten her hair and tiara before she headed up the aisle!

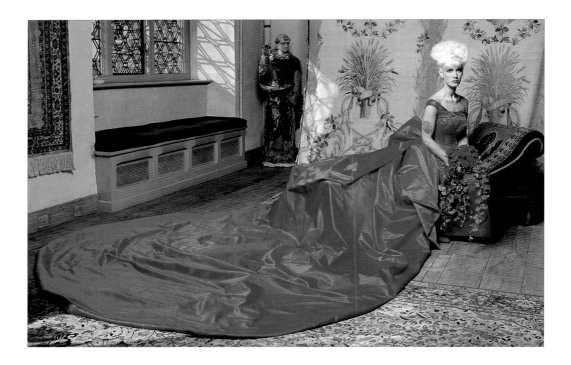

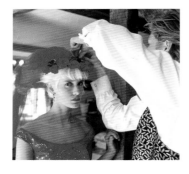

*Red roses and a scarlet dress …
the natural choice of wedding
outfit for Paula Yates.*

Somebody who has always had very definite ideas about
how she likes to look is Paula Yates, and this was no less
true of her wedding day. She is not only a client but one
of my great friends. I met her when she was seventeen
and have been doing her hair ever since. At that time,
around 1979, she had wild, bleached white hair. I think
we hit it off because I understood the spirit of how she
likes to look. She was young and vibrant and I was the
first hairdresser who didn't tut-tut about the bleach or
warn her of the dangers of split ends. You have to
understand what the client is about – this was the look
Paula wanted and nobody was going to change her mind.
She's always had her own ideas and style, and I work with
her on that. Maybe we don't always agree but we still get
on tremendously. She's changed her colour a couple of
times – she went red at one stage, not thanks to me! –
but now she's back to pale blonde again. No peroxide
now, though. We use a high-lift tint, which is gentler, and
she has exceptionally healthy hair. Of course I did her
wedding – a fantastic affair. She looked amazing in a
scarlet dress by Jasper Conran. Only Paula would
consider getting married in red.

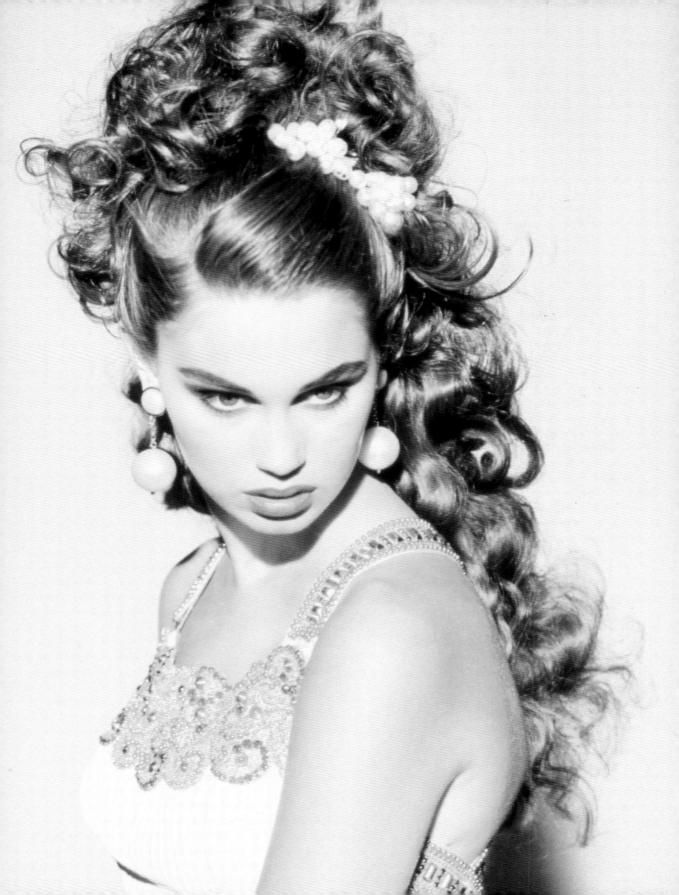

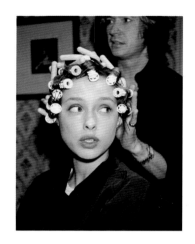 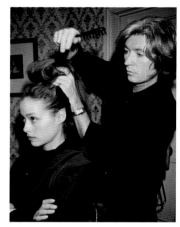 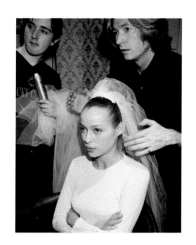

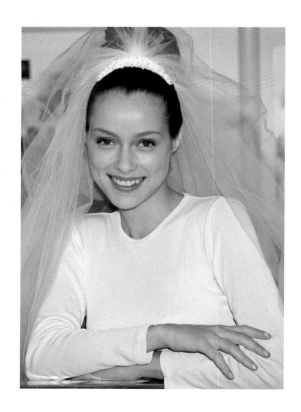

N I C O L E ' S   W E D D I N G

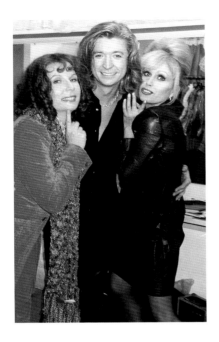

With Edina and Patsy, discussing Saffy's wedding-day hair for the final episode of Absolutely Fabulous.

Many a bride gets nervous. She wants this to be a day to remember but she occasionally veers towards boring hair. Yet there isn't a better time to plan and tackle a whole new style if that's what you want – you're going to be the star attraction, after all. But plan it well in advance with your hairdresser so that everything works together – your dress, headdress, hairstyle and confidence. I did Saffy's hair for her TV wedding on *Absolutely Fabulous*. It was great fun for Julia Sawalha, who played Saffy. Saffy was never a fashion victim like her mother, but she decided on a fashionable hairdresser for her wedding and it became one of the running jokes of the episode. In the end Saffy, or rather Julia, looked stunning – traditional but modern.

A more recent TV wedding I worked on was the Renault Clio advertisement. This was shrouded in secrecy. Everyone worked in isolation and no-one knew whom Nicole was to marry. The agency told us they were shooting three different endings and wanted two different looks for the actress Estelle Skornik. She was to wear a very pretty, young, summer wedding dress with a veil. I chose two looks, as far apart as they could be. For the first take I curled her hair in a long, loose, romantic style. For the second take I swept it back into a smooth knotted chignon – very French and very chic. I was thrilled to discover when the ad went out that they had chosen the chignon. And, no, I didn't know that she was going to run off with Bob Mortimer – I wasn't asked to do his hair.

When Amanda De Cadenet married John Taylor from Duran Duran, she went for a big change in her hair. Both Amanda and John had been clients for a long time. Amanda and I had discussed the change beforehand, and when I was getting her ready for the wedding I cut her the fringe we'd talked about. Only once it was done, she hated it! It looked great but that's no help if the bride doesn't like it. I thought I'd lost a client for ever and when she didn't come back I knew I had. But eight months later she returned. And the funny thing is that she's mostly worn styles with a fringe ever since.

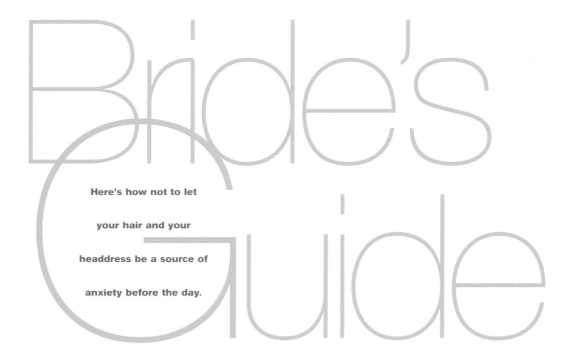

Bride's Guide

Here's how not to let your hair and your headdress be a source of anxiety before the day.

● Once you've chosen your dress and headdress, let your hairdresser into the secret. It's our job to help you look your best and we need the full picture.

● Have several appointments before the big day so that you can try out a few different ways of styling your hair and wearing your headdress. Make your appointments for the end of your working day or a work-free day – you don't want to have to go back to work looking as if you're off to a party. That way you'll also have a few hours of getting used to the style and seeing how stable it is.

● Tiaras are popular again, and even the lightest ones need careful anchoring with pins, plaits and hairpieces. During your practice sessions, give your hair a vigorous shaking to make sure the tiara stays put. A lot is demanded of a bride. For a start, everyone will want to kiss you and someone's hat is going to come into contact with your piece of hair engineering. Small bridesmaids occasionally need encouragement and you'll find yourself bending down to do so – it makes a great picture so long as your tiara's not sliding off. And there's no knowing what stray bits of a tree, a car, a pew or a table are going to lock on to your veil and give it a good tug.

- If you want to change your hairstyle, make sure you have discussed every aspect of it with your hairdresser beforehand. If you want to change your colour, do it a little in advance. This gives you time to get used to it and to make any necessary adjustments.

- If you want a light perm for extra body have that done in advance too – say two to three weeks beforehand, but not at the same time as having colour done.

- If you have a long veil, practise walking with it. One of my clients covered her bedroom floor, stairs and hall with sheets while she walked through the house keeping her head up. Another got a roll of very fine polythene from her dry-cleaners and cut the exact length of her veil from it. She wore it at every possible practice opportunity.

- Have at least one practice run for your make-up. Involve your hairdresser so that he can make adjustments to your hair if need be – it will only be something like tweaking a fringe to give more emphasis to your eyes. It all helps to make you feel great on your wedding day.

- Try not to look worried every time you try on your headdress. Smile, and you'll look better and feel massively more confident.

- If you are wearing a hat, give your hairdresser a chance to see it and work with it before the wedding – not on the day!

- Finally, if your hairdresser comes to your house to do your hair on the day of the wedding, do let him know in advance if you want him to do a quick style on your mum or grandma so that he allows himself time or brings somebody else along.

Boys Zone

Men, and British men in particular, have come rather late on to the caring-for-their-looks scene. A quick shampoo (often with a bar of soap) followed by a doggy shake of the head and a rub with the towel used to be all the notice they took of their hair – apart, of course, from a perfunctory trim every so often. But over the time I've been working as a hairdresser I've seen things change dramatically – men now perm, colour, highlight and restyle their hair whenever the mood or the fashion takes them.

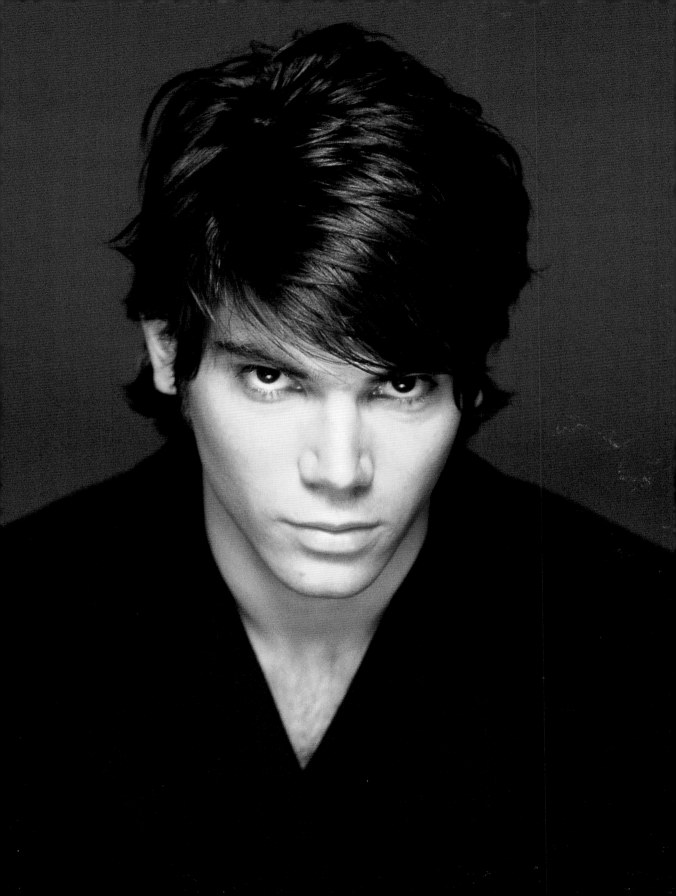

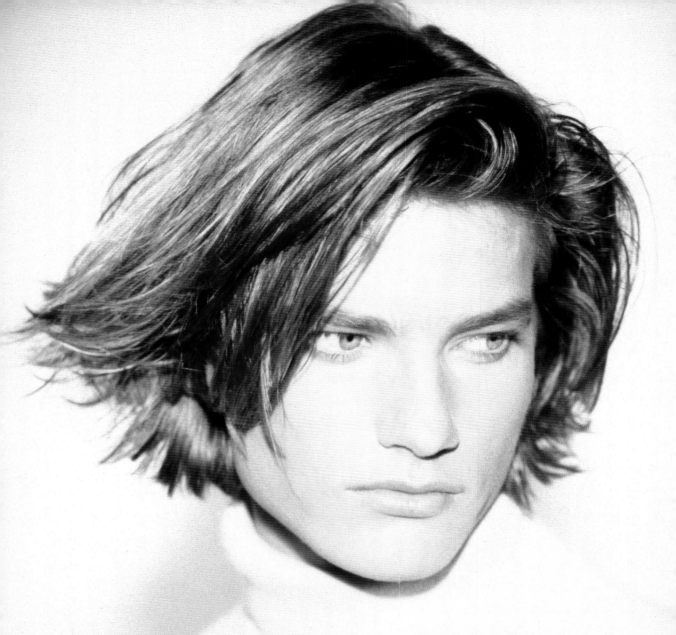

Men's styles haven't always been conservative. If you go back through the centuries, there have been some dramatic looks – from Renaissance princes to Cavaliers and Regency exquisites. But in the twentieth century, during the Twenties, Thirties and Forties, men's styles became very conservative. The only options were a bit of pomade here, a different parting there, and that was it.

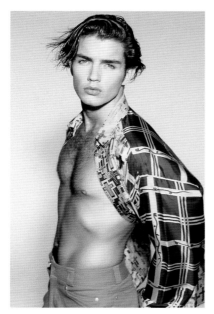

Matthew Marsden before he appeared in Coronation Street.

Things began to change during the Fifties. There was a rebellious feeling around, some pushing of boundaries. Maybe it was that post-war feeling of confidence. Tony Curtis was the first to sport one of the great twentieth-century men's hairstyles, the one that evolved into the DA (duck's arse, if you didn't know!). Before him there were just the three Ss – short, simple and slicked back, à la Rudolf Valentino, Clark Gable and James Stewart. This was a rakish quiff, whooshed and brilliantined and copied by men all over the world. Teddy Boys were the ones who really took it to heart – or to head – and there are great pictures from the Fifties showing guys in drapes, tight trousers, brothel creepers and those extravagant quiffs and DAs. This was the first time in decades that men had had the confidence to let their hair grow a little longer and, funnily enough, it caused more outrage than their dandified dress.

Of course this hairstyle led directly to the looks of two of the great twentieth-century male icons: James Dean and Elvis. While Dean had a shorter, cleaned-up version of the Tony Curtis with short sideburns to accompany the quiff, Elvis had the full monty – the DA, the slicked quiff, dangerously long sideburns and half a ton of brilliantine. Suddenly the world changed – it was one man, his music, his hips and his hair, and a revolution began. For the first time music and fashion became intertwined and a marriage was made that's still unbroken. It's as powerful today as it was then.

Alongside this, another type of American power was beginning to influence the rest of the world: the Harvard/Ivy League preppy look. Short hair and clean-cut looks full of thrust and ambition that would produce more millionaires, billionaires and zillionaires than in any other country on earth.

For the young and impressionable it was rock 'n' roll that changed everything, particularly the way men saw themselves. Our role models were musicians. They were the ones having a great time on stage, making loads of money and being pursued by girls – who wouldn't want a part of that action? Give me the haircut and I might get lucky! Since the rock 'n' roll days the great influences have been the Beatles' mop top, Jim Morrison's long poetic locks, Jagger's heavy fringe, Bowie in every guise, Bryan Ferry's matinee-idol style, the Sex Pistols' dramatic punk look, Spandau Ballet's glamorous New Romanticism, right through to Oasis and the retro-modern Brit pop scene.

Compared to the dangerous swagger of Elvis, it's extraordinary how clean-cut the following pop phenomenon was. Along came the Beatles with their shiny, bouncy heads of hair. But this was a style that changed the world. Suddenly, hair, which until then had been combed, slicked or swept back, was coming forward. It was still short at the sides and back but it was longer and heavier on top. The Beach Boys had their own variation with the heaviness going to the sides, but the pivotal change had already happened.

From then on it became a bit more Bohemian. Hair began to get longer – groups like the Stones exemplified this – and within a couple of years men's looks began to be much more flamboyant. The style leaders took their influences from everywhere: a bit of Afro, a bit of dandyism, a touch of art deco, a splash of the peacock. Old army jackets were mixed with washed-out jeans, florals and bright colours. It was the start of psychedelia and with the costumes of many extraordinary colours came hair as hippy as possible to balance them. The hippy element lasted through the early Seventies, transmuted into a sort of careless drop-out mood. It was all San Francisco and flower children, yet it was a very contrived fashion. Sure all the blokes had long hair, but with it they had exaggerated whiskers, long sideburns and mutton chops that hadn't seen the light of day for sixty-odd years.

And then feathering arrived. Shorter layers throughout a long style, with short layers on the top and sides and longer layers in the nape and below the ears. Practically every man in the country had it in one form or another.

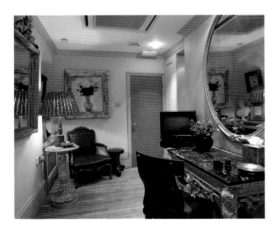

The walls of the salon VIP room could tell many stories about celebrities, supermodels and royalty. My lips will, of course, remain sealed.

For sheer style and confidence it's impossible to beat David Bowie. From the spiky Ziggy days to the smooth elegance of today he's always looked fantastic. One of my stylists – another David – does Bowie's hair, but when he's on holiday I have stood in. I've done his hair a few times and he's the easiest guy in the world to work on and to talk to. Bowie is very popular with the staff: he makes no fuss, no demands – but when I did his hair I took him to the VIP room because I wanted to maintain his privacy. When we were designing the salon I always knew I wanted a VIP room, simply to offer it to clients who are either fed up with too much attention or need some privacy. Of course, it was necessary for security purposes when I began to style the Duchess of York's hair. And if a client wants a new look for a particular film, promotion or tour they might not want to go public with it until the launch – so a VIP room is vital then to keep the new look a secret. There's a separate entrance to the VIP room, which means a client who wants privacy doesn't have to go through the main salon.

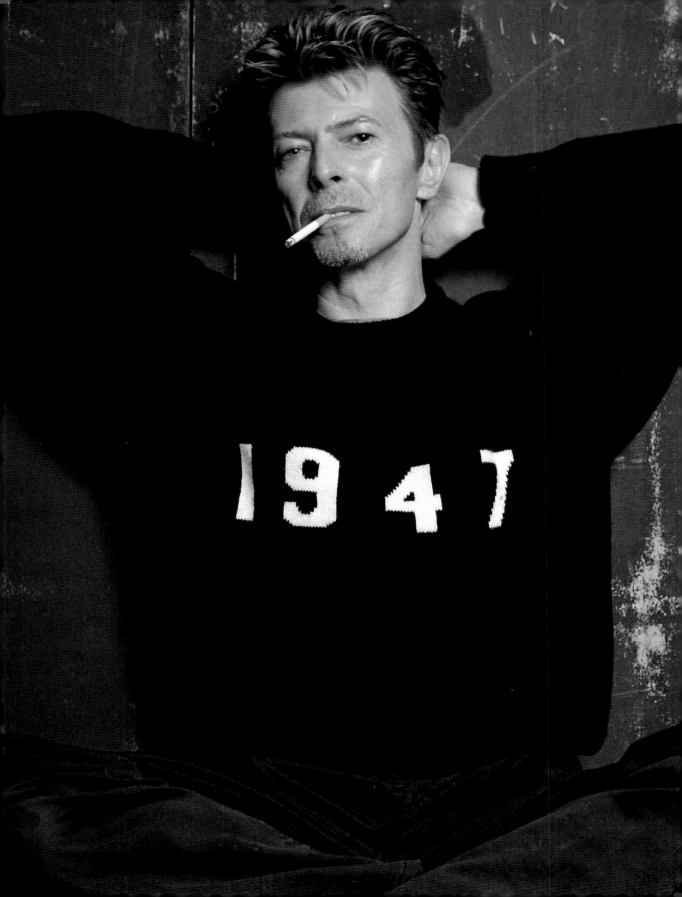

Around 1972 another major change in men's style took place, largely brought about by people such as Bryan Ferry. Whereas David Bowie had turned his looks into almost an art form, Ferry affected how the guys in the street, or more particularly in the clubs, wanted to look. Men went back to short hair, but for the first time it had splashes of colour in it – seriously fake colour. But it was the return of the haircut that was so image-shattering after years of free-flowing styles. And the cut was the wedge – heavy at the front and short everywhere else. Every soul boy from here to wherever had one. It was slick, it was sharp and it went with the fantastically sexy Anthony Price suits with the double-zipped crotch.

So in the early Seventies we saw concurrent styles, from the long-haired hippy variety through to glam rock, while short hair was making its comeback thanks to *The Great Gatsby* and Bryan Ferry. The Seventies also saw the start of the raw element of punk, which got stronger as we progressed through the decade. Punk, from a hair point of view, was very influential. It freed and fed people's imaginations. It was the first time hairstyles could defy gravity without resorting to wigs. This gave rise to the spiky Sid Vicious style alongside the Mohicans and vibrant colour – even more interesting was that it was happening more with men's hair than with women's. Barriers were broken down and the ground laid for the New Romantics in the early Eighties.

Over the years I've worked quite a lot with Duran Duran. Two of my clients are Yasmin Le Bon and Julie Ann Rhodes – both of whom I knew long before they met their respective husbands. And it was because of some styles and wigs I did for Anthony Price that I got to influence the styles worn by Nick Rhodes and the rest of the band.

The band were keen on their looks and their image and they all had both the style and the confidence to carry it off. Nick was a great stylist and with that first image I did for him he looked amazing – it's shown in a lot of pictures. It was great fun working with him, if a little exhausting. He completely reversed his day to everyone else's. He'd sleep long into the daylight hours and be up most of the night. I'd go round to

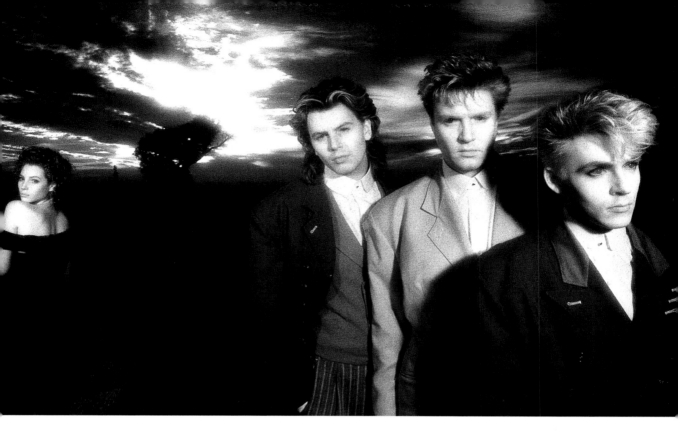

I travelled miles in a van with Duran Duran, Christy Turlington and photographer John Swannell to get this fantastic album cover shot. The boys took so long getting their hair, make-up and outfits right that we nearly lost the light.

his house at nine o'clock at night and we'd work on ideas until three or four in the morning. Then I'd go home for a short sleep before pitching up at the salon or a studio for a full day's work. But I wouldn't have missed it for anything. Duran Duran had a great image and worked almost as hard at maintaining that as they did at their music. In the end I did the whole group's hair.

The early Eighties was a fantastically exciting
time in my working life. The floodgates
opened. Everything that had once applied only
to women's hair now applied to men's – any
technique, any treatment, any style. Many of
the styles were almost unisex – long at the
back, shorter at the sides, layered at the top
and front – a real 'do'. To add even more
drama a lot of blond was in use, either all over
or in great thick chunks. For the first time men
began to use hairspray to keep their 'do' in
place, and then they began to experiment with
make-up too. Steve Strange, a real style guru,
was a client for quite some time, and he was a
great experimenter.

I suppose it was obvious that after such a fun time the pendulum would swing back
again. Sure enough, with the settling in of Thatcher's Britain we went back to short,
sober, conservative hair. These were the years of the suits – be they Armani, Next or
Boss. It was the time of the city boys: lunch was for wimps with everyone trying to get
their act together and make some money. There was no time for dressing, no time for
experiments – this was serious. Men had hair that needed just a shower plus a little bit
of gel, and fashions they could put together with their eyes closed: suits, shirts, ties.
The Masters of the Universe were not interested in how they looked. They were
interested in what they earned, hoping that in the end that would have more pulling
power than a feathery curl. For me it was a boring time for men's hair.

When the revival of long hair began in earnest, my own hair was very long. I'd seen
the style on my travels in California. It coincided with Calvin Klein putting a long-
haired model onto a giant billboard in Times Square, New York. I found myself
pulled out from behind the blow-dryer and shown as an example of what men with
long hair looked like, how they should look after it and what they should do with it.
All this was by chance. My hair grows incredibly fast and at this time I just let it grow.
I didn't have a single trim for two and a half years – in spite of the fact that I always
advise my clients to have a regular trim during a growing phase!

Now is a great time for men's hair. Anything goes. If you want it long that's fine because it can still look cool, medium length is not a problem in the style stakes, and if you want to be seriously cropped and short there's always the George Clooney.

When it comes to looking after hair, men have different priorities from women. Our main concern is hanging on to what we have! So men are often more concerned about the health of their hair than its look. Until a cure is discovered for baldness, it's a fact of hormones that men will lose hair. My view is that it's better to be dignified about this than to do a Bobby Charlton with the wisps we have left. Much better to go for the chop and keep it short. Tony Blair's recently done this – instead of sweeping back long thinning bits he's had the front cut very short. It looks grown-up and elegant and even though I had nothing to do with it we did at least keep it in the family. My sister-in-law, Frances, did it.

Neither do men want to spend too much time on their hair. They want whatever style they have to be easy. They don't want to spend time blow-drying, and perish the thought that they should put a roller in – that's why the George Clooney is so popular, along with the styles the guys from *Friends* have. Unsurprisingly, the time-saving two-in-one shampoo and conditioner products are popular with men. I've developed a whole new range specially for men. We produce more natural oil and consequently get more dandruff than women do, and we don't always have the patience to deal with it. Men want effective products that are quick and easy to use and that will keep their scalps clean and healthy. When they want texture and definition they opt for a gel or a soft wax rather than any other styling product. My new men's range addresses all this.

We've come a long way from the short back and sides of the early decades of this century. In many ways we have to thank those – mostly actors, rock 'n' rollers and style icons – who broke the mould and allowed men to have the same freedom with hair as women.

I have great respect for performers. They have to give so much of themselves – even when they don't feel like it. Whether on stage or on television they give of themselves, plus all their energy, while at the same time looking their best and pretending not to mind the criticism. It takes great guts. I first became aware of this when I was working with Lulu. I saw at first-hand how hard she worked and what performing means. It also gave me a chance to see what hair needed to be like to withstand the rigours of being on stage, on tour and on show all the time. I even styled her wig for *Peter Pan*!

Rock stars still influence the way people want to look, so looking after their hair is a great way of seeing moods and fashions change. And one thing I've learned from working with some of the most famous bands in the world, not to mention the world's best models, is that everybody needs a confidence boost at some stage. Even the most famous faces and the top singers feel better about themselves if they know they're looking their best. And the same goes for all of us. I know that whoever comes into my salon feeling low or fed up will go home looking better and feeling great. Everyone's confidence increases when they are happy with the way they look – especially when their hair feels right.

Staff and clients in my salon are used to seeing well-known faces, but it was amazing how many people completely lost their cool the day Brad Pitt and Gwyneth Paltrow came in to get their colour touched up!

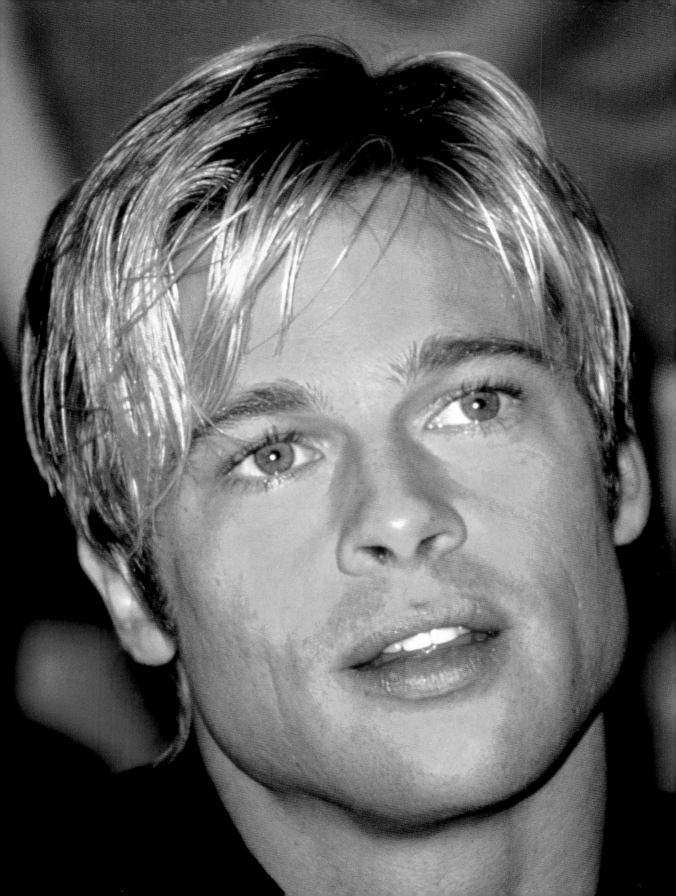

THE POWER OF SEDUCTION

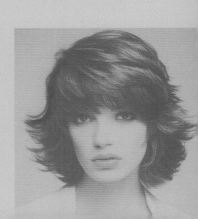

The sort of hair I like and the sort of hair I'm known for are one and the same thing. I like hair to look *sexy* but not *tarty*, with a good finish and a glossy sheen. It should be well groomed, but it shouldn't look as if its owner's spent all day at the hairdresser's. There's nothing seductive about somebody who's tried too hard. And if there's a Nicky Clarke look, then that's the basis of it.

Hair's

been sexy since time began. You only have to look at medieval paintings of Adam and Eve in the Garden of Eden. Before the apple it was unashamed nakedness, while afterwards Eve tried to cover herself with her hair. Delilah wanted to make sure of Samson's presence and love, so what did she do? She cut off his hair. Paintings and literature throughout the centuries have gloried in the power and beauty of hair, from Botticelli's *Venus*, whose golden hair was her only adornment, to *The Rape of the Lock*, where men went into a frenzy for just one curl. Lady Godiva was able to declare her love and support for her husband, in spite of Peeping Tom, by wearing just her hair. And Rapunzel was able to escape for love by using hers.

Poets, painters, lovers – you name it, they've all had something to say about our crowning glory. It's been pretty powerful stuff along the way. Was it really surprising that one of the first things young girls did on entering a convent was have their hair cut? So provocative and arousing was it thought to be. And then to increase the seductive powers of those outside the convent walls, their hair was sold to make wigs for the rich. Even today some cultures and religions find hair so erotic and suggestive that it has to be hidden beneath veils and shawls.

There's something very sensual and seductive about freshly washed, shining hair – the way it falls and feels and smells. It's one of the first things people notice about you, along with your face, and it's one of the things they remember. Often it's used as a means of identifying a person. How often do we say the one with long hair, or the blonde, or even the guy with the crop? And because it's one of our most easily identifiable assets, hair can cause us real angst when we can't do a thing with it. A bad hair day can be caused by anything from a hormonal blip to a late night. No matter how we dry, style, fiddle, scrape back or cover with a hat, it doesn't do any good. *Nobody* has ever felt sexy on a bad hair day. How can you feel good when you're sure you don't look good?

But when your hair is glossy, gleaming and healthy-looking, you feel as though you could conquer the world.

Very few people have glossy, gleaming hair naturally and effortlessly, but I've been lucky enough to work with a few of them. Yasmin Le Bon has the most fantastic hair. It's Iranian hair, and the reflection in it is like glass; we really had to work at it to mess it up a bit. Even perfection must get boring after a while! I think that's why Yasmin fancied a change of look and style. We'd been gradually taking it shorter and shorter

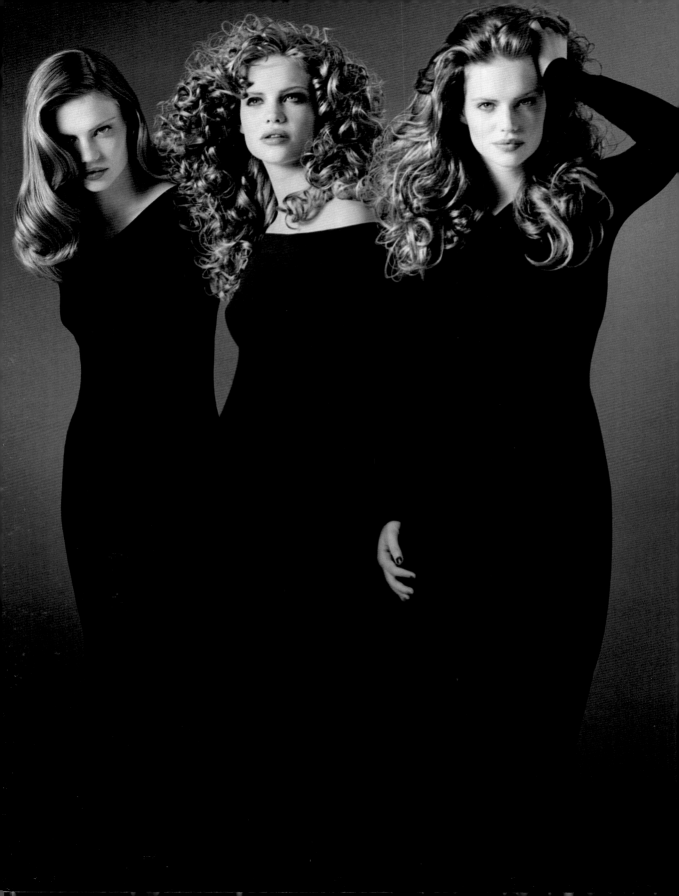

until one day we decided to go for it and chop it off. First of all we made it blonde with great lights and wide streaks of colour, and then I cut it in a very choppy fashion with texture and depth. It was probably the only time grunge was made glamorous – because it (and she) still looked fantastically sexy.

Possibly the most fantastic hair I've ever done is Maria Shriver's, Arnold Schwarzenegger's wife. I always do her hair when they're in England. She has seriously glossy, very thick, slightly wavy hair. There's a type of American hair that's a combination of a middle-European and a Native American heritage. This hair is big and glossy and thick and you see it as much in downtown LA as in uptown New York, as well as all across the States. The sort of hair that Christie Brinkley, Julia Roberts and Cindy Crawford have – well, that's the type Maria Shriver, has but she has it in spades. You can do almost anything with it: style it straight, wavy, curly, make it tousled, put it back, put it up or merely tweak it, and it just shines through. Even better is that she's extremely professional, knows exactly how she wants to look and is very good to work with. She's a television presenter in the US and understands perfectly what suits her and what's right for her image. That sort of self-knowledge is very seductive in a man or woman.

Great American hair has played a big part in influencing the way we've looked over the years. Some of the sexiest hairstyles of this century have come from across the Atlantic, either in movies or on TV, and they've changed the way women have wanted to portray themselves. From Louise Brooks onwards, women have wanted a share of that seductive power. In the great glamour days of Hollywood you saw the influence at its peak. To begin with there were all the great blondes: the platinum babes from Jean Harlow to Marilyn Monroe. Harlow was the most overtly sexy, while Monroe was just heart-stoppingly seductive. Monroe didn't have great hair – you couldn't with the amount of peroxide she needed to keep it that shade – but she knew exactly how to make it work for her: fluffy, wispy and vulnerable. With a hairdresser constantly on duty she'd have her hair done twice a day – but the great thing about her was that it looked its best when it was slightly dishevelled and not too done.

But it was in the Forties, with all those film parts for strong manipulative women, that the seductive power of hair was at its zenith. There was Joan Crawford's roll – tight but with enough curve in it to let you know it could be unleashed at the drop of a diamond or two. Bette Davis's fringe was lethal – no wonder Americans call fringes 'bangs'. Veronica Lake's come-hither wavy pageboy is a perennial favourite. Hair that falls across and almost hides one eye gives a woman a certain knowingness that's incredibly sexy. It's a style that gets adapted by each generation: Lauren Bacall had her version in the Fifties, Shirley Eaton, the *Goldfinger* girl, had it during the Sixties, Bryan Ferry took it up in the Seventies, Jerry Hall emerged in the Eighties with her version which she still wears to devastating effect, and the original has just re-emerged on Kim Basinger in *LA Confidential*. It's a killer combination of gentle waves, serious shine and downright naughtiness. No wonder it's retained its popularity.

As the Sixties came to an end a new style began to emerge. The bouffants and beehives started to relax and come down and were replaced by their polar opposite: uncoiffed, natural-looking hair almost childlike in its lack of guile and style. It was long, straight and shiny. Or rather that's what it was supposed to be. Simple though it may sound, it took for ever to get right – but more than anything it led the revolution in hair which we all benefit from now.

As the Seventies rolled in, the real change in attitudes in this country and across the world became more and more obvious. Hair and hairdressing was just one small part of that change. Women now have a collective dose of amnesia about how to dress their own hair. Not so long ago, every woman knew how to set it, pin it, wave it and curl it. Women did their own hair and each other's. Then freedom beckoned. There was a new movement around, a new sense of youth and freedom, and a new style.

The revolution in hairdressing was brought about by two men, both in London: Vidal Sassoon and Leonard. Vidal was the engineer and draughtsman, Leonard was the sculptor. Vidal created the five-point cut: sharp, straight, sexy and very modern. Leonard created shapes and softness: he gave the sharp points and edges a freeflow dimension, a sensual quotient. Hairdressing in London is still carried out in these two schools of thought and traces its influences back to these two salons. My training was at Leonard's, which is why my styling has always veered towards the tousled rather than the taut, the soft rather than the sharp.

Hair Freedom

What these two men did was as liberating for the wearer as was the move from stockings to tights. They introduced Hair Freedom. Until then if a woman went to the hairdresser her style was meant to last for the whole week – she didn't even wash it. Many women went to bed wearing rollers: really uncomfortable ones with pins sticking into their skulls. But with the cuts and movement now coming through, rollers and pin curls were thrown out and all you really needed was a dryer, a wide-toothed comb and a round brush to celebrate the birth of the blow-dry. If you asked a woman now to put in a Velcro roller while she's getting ready, the chances are she'd think you were crazy – even if you were only suggesting a quick fix.

In some instances a Denman brush was all that was necessary. In others a piece of brown paper and an iron were called into play for those who couldn't get straight, straight hair without ironing it.

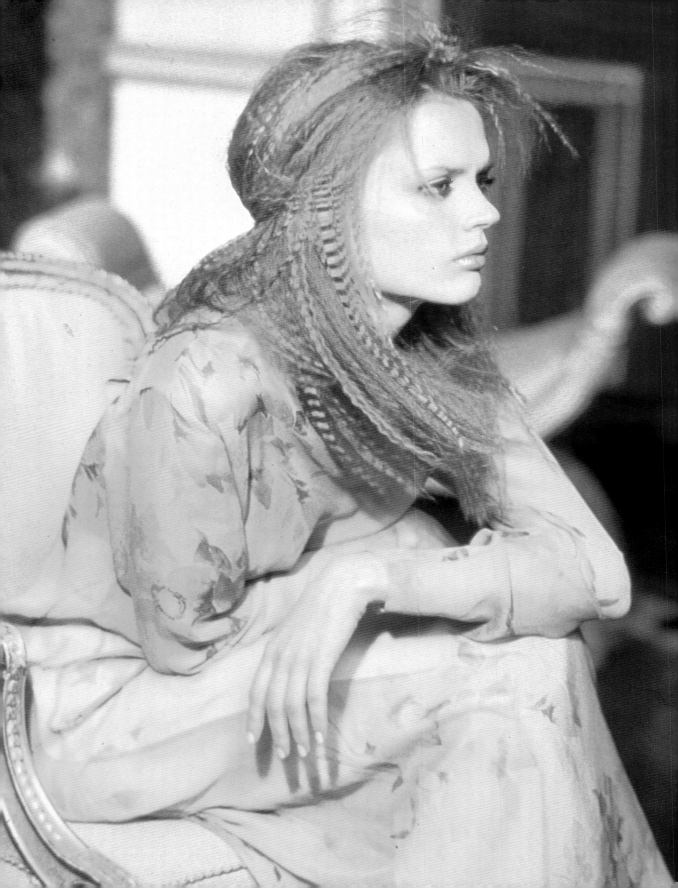

Everyone who had long hair wanted to look like Julie Christie and Marianne Faithfull, while those who had short hair wanted to look like Twiggy. It was the child/woman style, sensuous rather than blatantly sexy. Hairdressing – and hairdressers – got a real boost in the image stakes when the movie *Shampoo* was released with superstud Warren Beatty in the lead role, rampant with a blow-dryer. His love interest was every man's fantasy: Julie Christie.

The late Seventies and early Eighties were a great time for me. I was developing all kinds of skills and learning a heck of a lot. I still worked in the salon. I was doing a lot of work for the monthly magazines – covers and before-and-afters. Even when I was working on fashion sessions, I'd always tried to give the models a style they'd be happy with and want to keep once the shoot was over. I wanted them to feel good about the style as well as making a great picture. But the stakes weren't high for them. They could keep the look or wash it out. The women who'd come for makeovers had invested their hopes and dreams in being chosen for a magazine makeover and you had to make them look and feel terrific.

I still love the challenge of makeovers, which is why they are such an important part of my *This Morning* slot. Every week I get the chance to observe a shift in attitude in a makeover subject when she sees the potential a better hairstyle gives her. In most cases it's not a major change of style. It's just that for a change someone has looked at her, talked to her and, most important of all, listened to her to find out what she wants and what suits her best. Helping someone feel more confident, and consequently more sexy and attractive, gives me a real buzz.

At the same time as all these magazine sessions I was also doing some of the wildest hairdressing I've ever done. One of my best friends is Chris Duffy. I met him through working with his dad, Duffy, the great Sixties photographer. Chris and I did a lot of sessions together – practice sessions as well as special things for our own portfolios. At this time, around 1978, he was living with one of the girls from Hot Gossip and we did all the group's pictures. They were fantastic and really experimental with their looks. Sarah Brightman went along with much of the experimenting too, though she was more conservative than the other girls. However, there'd never been a group of dancers like them. They were young, fantastic-looking, sexy and very radical. We put some amazing looks together. I gave them multi-coloured hair, then wild extensions, then a mixture of the two. Often we would work all through the night doing their photographs.

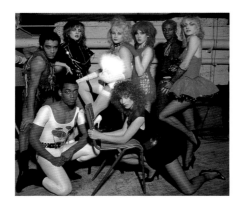

*Hot Gossip – in the wild
and zany Seventies.*

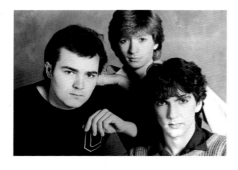

*Three young dudes perfecting their
styles and techniques. Yours truly at
the back, photographer Chris Duffy on
the left, and make-up artist Stevie
Hughes on the right. We all had great
fun on those Hot Gossip sessions.*

I was passionate about their image and looks
but all the while I was developing my own style
too. I always had a slightly romantic feel for
hair. Even when we did the wildest style with
Hot Gossip there was never a hard edge. The
styles were striking and occasionally avant-
garde but they were never ugly.

Gradually the Nicky Clarke look developed
through a mixture of makeovers and studio
work. I was pretty unique in that I still, in spite
of all the photographic work, continued to
work in the salon. Somehow I always knew that
I didn't want to lose my base. This is what
drove me, and in many ways still does. I think
the most difficult part of hairdressing is
coming up with something accessible but not
boring, something avant-garde but beautiful.
It's easy to do something wild but unwearable.

We've seen it recently in London with the
fashion shows and the whole Cool Britannia
thing. All the buyers and commentators have
been going around saying how wonderful, wild
and way ahead London is in fashion, and then
off they go to Milan, breathe a sigh of relief
and remark on how wearable the clothes are.
Well, I wanted the wearable tag mixed with the
wild so there'd never be any dullness. And
that's what I aimed for after the Hot Gossip
days: the job of producing styles that are
beautiful as well as wearable.

The key to really beautiful, sexy hair is hair that doesn't look preened and coiffed but
hair that's touchable. Hair that invites stroking and caressing. For this it has to look
clean, shiny and naturally well groomed. There's something really seductive about
women who are well groomed: they have an inner confidence that comes from a pride
in their appearance. I'm not talking about women who are obsessed with how they
look – that's a real turn-off. This has more to do with women who value themselves,
their attitudes and their presentation.

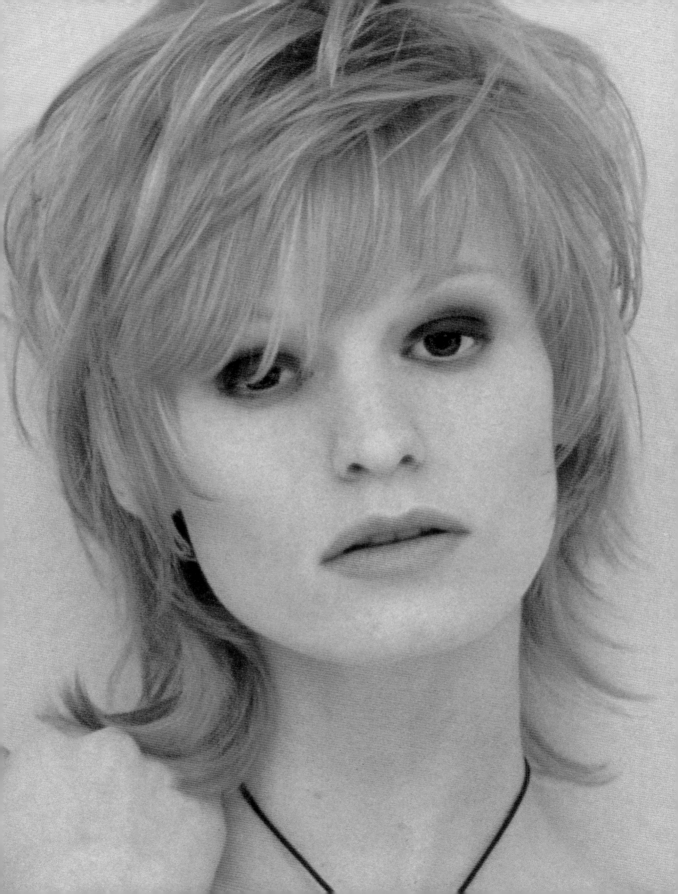

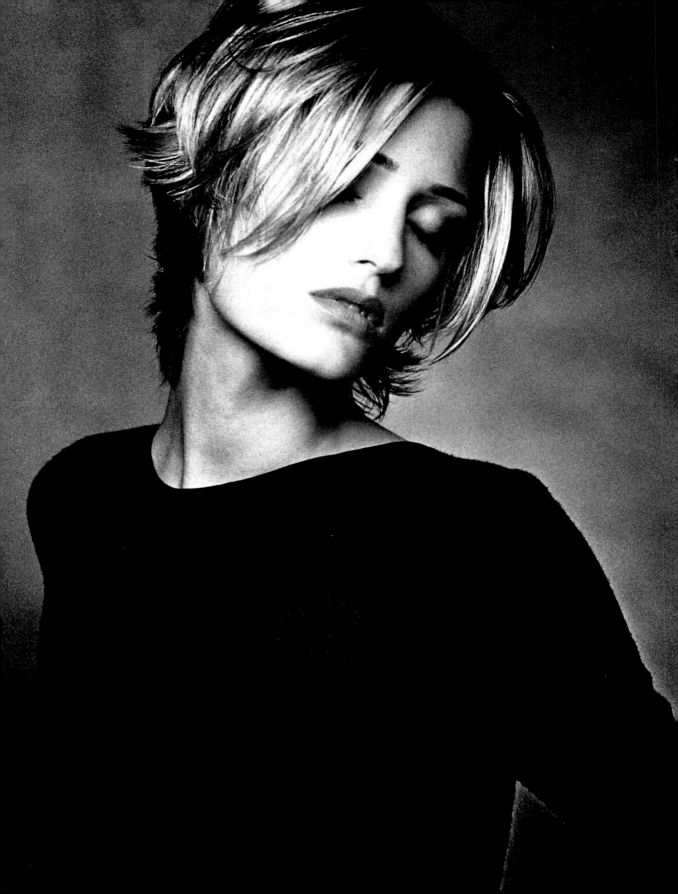

It's the difference between the woman who goes out and gets a whole designer wardrobe – the shoes, the bag, the dress, the coat, the lot – and the type of woman who chooses bits and pieces from different designers and adapts the look to suit her own style and her own wardrobe. With the designer-label woman it somehow always looks just a little contrived, as if she doesn't trust her own judgement and taste and allows the wardrobe to wear her. A woman who has a mind of her own and who knows what suits her evinces an effortless elegance.

This demands a confidence that until recently a lot of British women lacked – but they're catching up fast! The same attitude used to prevent British women spending too much time, care and attention, not to mention money, on how they looked. It's an attitude completely alien to French and American women, who think it only right and proper that they look after themselves and have massages and facials and manicures – not out of vanity but because they know they deserve it. New Yorkers, both men and women, think nothing of having a manicure in their lunch-break or a massage after work. Central Manhattan is awash with nail bars and beauty parlours and going to them is as easy and normal as going to the supermarket or the hairdresser's. And the more a woman is good to herself and values herself, the more alluring she can be.

Everybody at some point wants to make a strong statement about his or herself. You want to be noticed, to make a mark. For occasions such as this you need what I call Result Hair. I took the idea from Anthony Price, who in each collection always has a Result Dress: a real knock-'em-between-the-eyes frock. His clothes are sexy at the best of times but the result one is the knockout. When he is making a dress he builds it from the inside, concentrating on its foundation – the boning, the padding, the oomph. Once the structure is there the fabric can just be draped over – it's an astonishingly sexy look. Everybody who wears a result dress looks amazing – Jerry Hall, Marie Helvin, Lucy Ferry. I started to do a similar thing with hair. Result hair is built around the body in a style. Not so much so that it begins to look like a rigid 'hairdo', but just enough to have a foundation around which I add some shorter bits of hair, either in a fringe or little fronds that hit the face somewhere round the cheeks or mouth in a slight tumble. There's nothing static about it. It has enough movement to be touchable and it doesn't look as if it's just been done. Everything about it moves, yet every single rudiment of the style has been built in. In effect, it's hair with loads of body but enough style and movement for you to change it around without relying on sprays and holds.

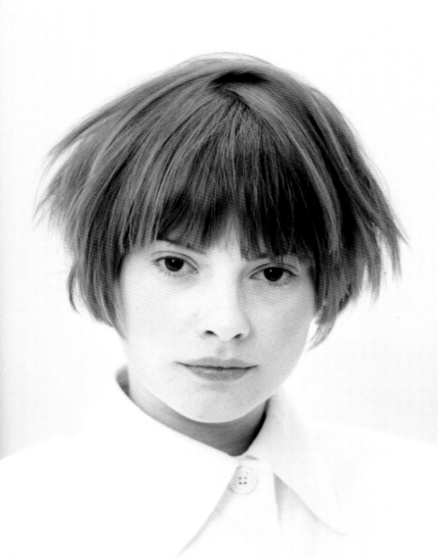

A woman who

has a mind of

her own and

who knows

what suits her

evinces an

effortless

elegance.

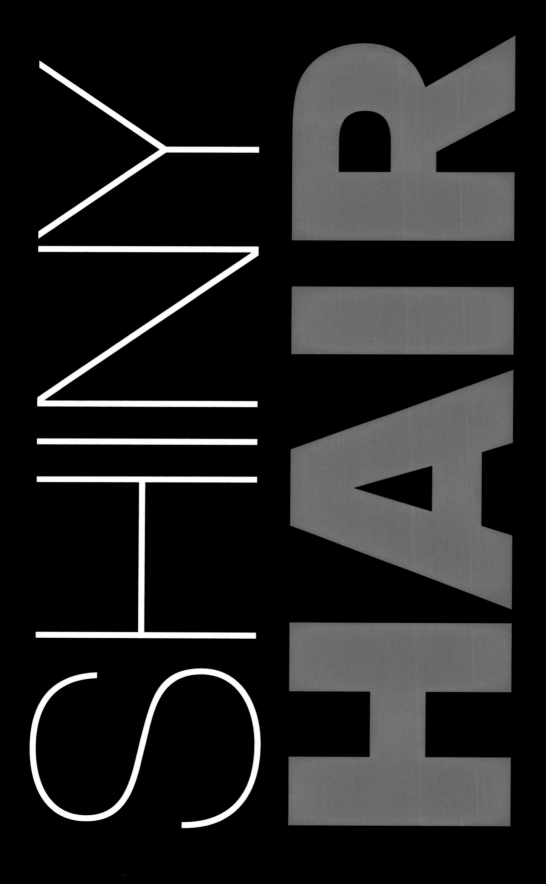

ONE OF THE MOST SENSUAL ASPECTS OF HAIR IS ITS TOUCHABILITY. IT HAS TO LOOK INVITING AND FOR THAT IT HAS TO HAVE SHINE AND SWING. EVEN THE SHORTEST OF STYLES MUST HAVE A SENSE OF MOVEMENT ABOUT THEM. SELINA SCOTT'S VERY SHORT STYLE WAS LOVED BY MEN; THEY THOUGHT IT SEXY. EVEN THOUGH IT WAS SHORT AT THE BACK AND SIDES IT HAD GREAT MOVEMENT AND A LOT OF SWING. WOMEN LOVED IT TOO. ANTHEA TURNER'S INSOUCIANCE IS INCREDIBLY ATTRACTIVE – HER HAIR ALWAYS HAS THAT SLIGHTLY RUFFLED LOOK WHICH, AGAIN, MEN LOVE. ANYTHING THAT SHINES CATCHES THE EYE – BE IT A DIAMOND OR A PIECE OF TIN – WHICH IS WHY SEXY HAIR HAS TO BE SHINY.

SHINY HAIR LOOKS HEALTHY, ATTRACTIVE, TOUCHABLE, DESIRABLE – AND THAT'S WHY EVERYBODY WANTS IT.

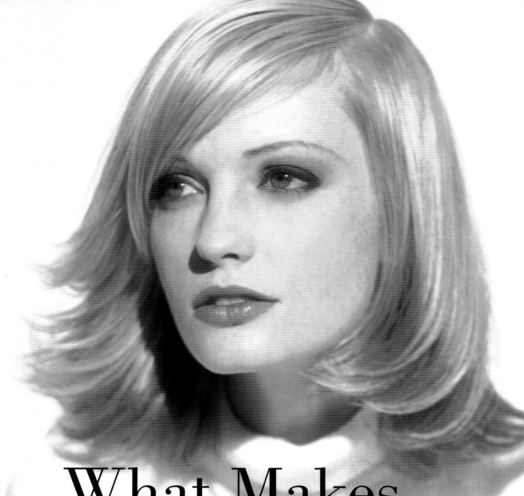

What Makes
Hair Shine

The surface of each individual hair must lie flat so that it can reflect the light. This surface – the cuticle – is made up of tiny overlapping scales like fish scales, which, when they are raised, damaged or broken off, give a rough finish to the hair that doesn't reflect the light. Consequently, the smoother the surface the better and deeper the shine. That's why curly hair never appears as shiny as straight hair. It's not necessarily damaged, but its surface is uneven because of the curls and so light doesn't reflect so highly from it.

GOING FOR MAXIMUM SHINE

Follow these guidelines and you'll be on the way to having the shiny, touchable hair you've always longed for.

- Shampoo frequently: dust and dirt take away the gloss.
- Keep your brush and comb scrupulously clean.
- Always use a conditioner and rinse thoroughly.
- Never brush wet hair: this can cause tangles as well as stretching the hair to breaking point.
- Use a wide-toothed comb on wet hair to de-tangle: never pull, and never start from the root. Always begin just above the tangle itself.
- For extra shine on curly hair you need to dry it straight, which requires a tight hold on the hair you're blow-drying. To keep both curl and shine you need to get more definition into the curl, either by letting it dry naturally, or by pin-curling or tonging it. Use products with frizz-control ingredients; my range has shampoo, conditioner, serum and balm, all of which help control the curl and frizz and add extra shine.
- Watch the angle of your dryer – the air should go down the hair shaft to help the cuticle stay flat.
- Give a shine boost by using a special serum that contains silicones for extra smoothness. In the Hairomatherapy range we have one for frizz control and one spray-on that's so light and fine it can be used on any hair type. A word of advice: you need only the minutest amount.

Finally, hair has to smell good. A whiff of stale tobacco or fried food is a real turn-off. When my wife Lesley and I were developing our own hair-care range we insisted upon great smells alongside the best possible ingredients. And that's one of the reasons why we are so keen on aromatherapy: the fragrances from the natural oils are so wonderful.

In the Hairomatherapy range our products include the fresh scents of lime, spearmint and sea kelp alongside the wholesomeness of jojoba, aloe vera and camomile mixed with the spiciness of bergamot, sage and rosemary next to the headiness of neroli, sandalwood and ylang ylang. But not all in the same jar! Each one is used for a specific purpose. For instance, jojoba for its moisturizing qualities, wheatgerm for strength and ylang ylang to soothe.

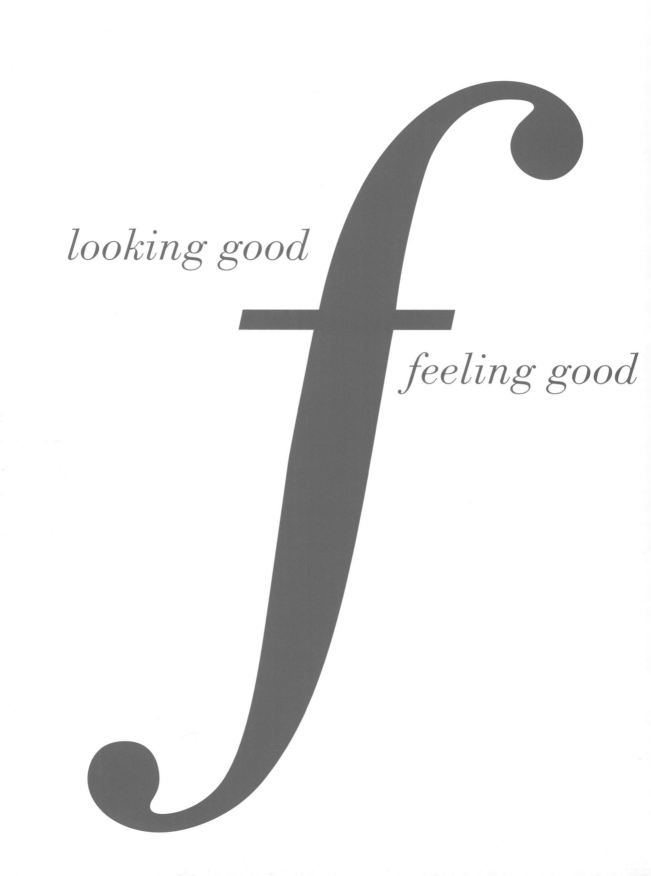

looking good

feeling good

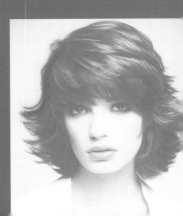

Everybody wants healthy, glossy, shining, bouncy hair and yet few of us spend much time thinking about how to get it and keep it. Most of us think that regular shampooing and conditioning is our contribution to healthy, shiny hair, and when hair begins to look dull and feel dry and strawlike we blame either the products we've been using or the person who does our hair. Each of these *may* have worsened the problem but in most cases we need to look to ourselves, how we treat and care for our hair and what we do to maintain its health.

There's an old saying that if your feet hurt it shows in your face. Well, if you are not in the peak of health, that shows in your hair too. Your hair reflects how you feel. If it's dull and lifeless, it's only revealing the state of your health. If it's glossy, full and shiny then it's reflecting the healthy body it adorns.

When your diet is poor and you're overstressed, hair can look lank and lifeless. If you're recovering from an operation, your hair won't be in peak condition: it will register that anaesthetics have been introduced into your body. If you're on prescription drugs or recovering from an illness your hair can lose its gloss and bounce. When a woman is pregnant and all her hormones are rattling around in perfect working order then both her skin and hair can sometimes bloom to perfection. However, trouble can start after pregnancy. Within the first week, hair loss begins. When new hair begins to grow back it does so quite prominently around the hairline and at the front. I can nearly always tell how old the baby is when I see the mother's hair.

Hormones play a major part in how our hair looks and behaves. In troublesome adolescence many young girls suffer from lank or greasy hair as well as from mood swings, acne and weight fluctuations. At the other end of the scale, during menopause, hair can be dull, dry and lifeless. Stress is another obstacle on the road to strong, healthy hair. Stress, or at least a certain amount of it, is necessary and can be good for us, but too much can lead to thin, lifeless hair.

So, if you want to know the state of someone's health, look at their crowning glory. Add to dull, lank and lifeless hair a dry and flaky scalp and we have work to do. Of course, when we're young, apart from the odd hormonal hiccup we tend not to worry too much about our health. But as we get older we begin to recognize the signs. Women know that the menstrual cycle can play havoc with their emotional wellbeing, and it doesn't take much imagination to see that it also has an effect on skin and hair. Men aren't so quick on the uptake. They only really begin to look at every aspect of their lives when they first start to lose their hair. I must admit it took me some time to recognize the impact of one's state of health. And the older I get, the more I realize how important it is to look after the whole body and the whole mind. I try to eat sensibly and maintain my weight. I go to the gym to work out and look after my shape. Part of it is vanity, of course, but much of it is also sound common sense.

It takes a lot of effort to keep looking good. I know because I've spent so much time working with models at photographic studios, on shoots and during fashion shows. Their looks are their livelihood so they are masters at improvement and maintenance. They are also among the first to know when some new research has revealed which vitamins and minerals are best for skin and hair because they travel so much and learn

BANNED!

This provocative advertising campaign won an award for the best campaign of the year – despite being banned by two national newspapers

TranSport *by* Nicky Clarke.

The Rules. 1 Remove clothing. 2 Remove partner's clothing. 3 Grab a pack of Nicky Clarke Sport Protein Shampoo from the new Sport range. 4 Massage into wet hair the rich, nutrifying combination of Vitamin E, Wheat protein and Pro Vitamin B5. 5 Rinse. 6 Enjoy. 7 Don't get carried away.

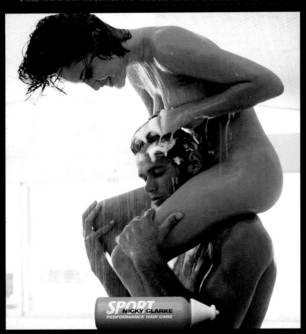

Synchronised Sport *by* Nicky Clarke.

The Rules. 1 Remove clothing. 2 Remove partner's clothing. 3 Grab a pack of Nicky Clarke Sport Wake Up Spa Shampoo from the new Sport range. 4 Massage into wet hair the invigorating combination of Green Tea Extract and Menthol. 5 Rinse. 6 Enjoy. 7 Altogether now ...

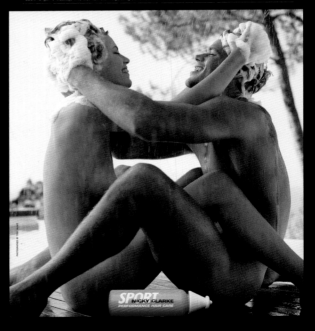

from the people they work with, who include some of the world's top beauty specialists and journalists. They know every faddy diet going and every exercise guru from Miami to Milan.

I've also learned a lot from my clients, many of whom are women who take great care of their health and their looks. They read voraciously and they know who are the experts on nutrition, exercise and stress relief. They have husbands and families whose health they are also passionate about. Anybody who spends a morning listening in at my salon could easily discover where their own diet and exercise regime is going wrong. I spend a lot of time and care on our in-salon menu because I need to cater for such informed clients. Besides ordinary coffees and teas we offer the decaffeinated variety, several tisanes, wholewheat bread, healthy salads and a choice of dressings.

Many people these days are very aware of what's good for them – even if they take no notice of it. Men, although latecomers to the health and fitness scene, have taken to it like the proverbial duck to water. Look at the phenomenal growth in men's magazines over the last few years, and the pages that are devoted to health, fitness and grooming routines. Most men I know cannot get enough information on how to improve their health.

We might be pretty knowledgeable these days, but we can still get it wrong. We might become a little too obsessive, a little too keen to get on to the latest diet and exercise bandwagon. All we need to do is channel this knowledge and information into a state of balance. A balanced lifestyle and a balanced diet. If you can get that sorted out you are well on the way to enjoying a healthy lifestyle – much of which will be reflected in your hair.

Food for Thought

We have been through so many fads and fashions about what constitutes a healthy diet that it's hardly surprising that we sometimes get confused. And there have been many times over the last twenty or so years when experts have got it wrong, or new research has caused them to change their minds. Then there are the commercial concerns of the vast food-manufacturing business. We've had the high-fibre fashion, we've lived through the high-cholesterol scares, abandoned fats of every type, forsworn sugars, eggs and red meats, dispensed with caffeine and sodium, been terrified by BSE scares and are still working our way through the minefields of overproduction and factory farming. There have been times in the past few years when all we felt we could eat were a handful of leaves and a few nuts – and even those only if you weren't allergic to them.

Somehow, in spite of all this knowledge, we're told we're the fattest and unhealthiest we've ever been as a nation. Running parallel with this are the growing numbers of young girls (and young men now too) with eating disorders. Some experts estimate that as many as 60 per cent of all teenage girls suffer, or will do at some time, from such a disorder.

My view is that the only way you can get through all of this is to fall back on the age-old rule of thumb that a little of what you fancy does you good. If you can have a reasonably balanced diet and take some form of exercise on a regular basis then at least you're in with a chance.

A well-balanced diet of some protein – meat or fish or cheese – some carbohydrate – potatoes or pasta or rice – and large helpings of fruit and vegetables, is mostly what we need. Far too few people eat enough fresh fruit and vegetables, but listening to both my clients and staff I know that many of us are trying to rectify this. I also know from the nutritionists and doctors I've worked with that we're also much more likely now to search out organically produced fruit and vegetables. We've listened to the warnings, read the signs and decided that we've had enough of pesticide-ridden foods. Those of us with children are made constantly aware of what we are doing, first to our own bodies and then to our countryside and environment, by not taking action on any or all of these fronts. Many of us have little green monsters in our midst watching our every mouthful and asking questions that could nearly put you off your breakfast!

FOODS HAIR LOVES

- Fresh fruits, particularly red and orange ones such as oranges, uglis, clementines, tangerines, grapefruit, pineapple, mangoes, papaya, apricots, peaches and black grapes.
- Salad vegetables: lettuce, baby spinach, watercress, rocket, tomatoes, avocadoes, cucumber and chicory.
- Vegetables: all the greens from cabbage to asparagus, plus red peppers, carrots, onions, cauliflower, courgettes, celery, leeks and broccoli.
- Wholegrains: brown rice, wholewheat pasta, wholemeal breads and porridge.

FOODS HAIR LIKES

- Protein: chicken, small portions of red meat, fish, especially oily varieties such as salmon, sardines and herring, and small helpings of hard cheeses and eggs.
- Pulses such as beans and lentils.
- Unsaturated fats such as cold-pressed olive and safflower oils; small amounts of butter.

FOODS HAIR WOULD RATHER YOU AVOIDED

- Saturated fats, anything processed, biscuits, cakes, chocolate and sugar, crisps, salted nuts, salted anything, creams, burgers, frankfurters and anything deep-fried.

DRINKS

- Water: lots, at least a litre and a half a day.
- Herbal or fruit teas. If you cannot do without caffeine, limit your intake to one or two cups of coffee or tea a day.
- Watch the alcohol – one or two glasses of wine maximum (red is better for your blood than white) or one glass of beer a day.
- Fruit juices: one or two glasses a day. Vegetable juices are even better; see below.
- Vegetable drinks such as carrot, celery, tomato or V8. Invest in a juicer and make your own – these are great for de-tox days.
- Avoid colas or other fizzy drinks.

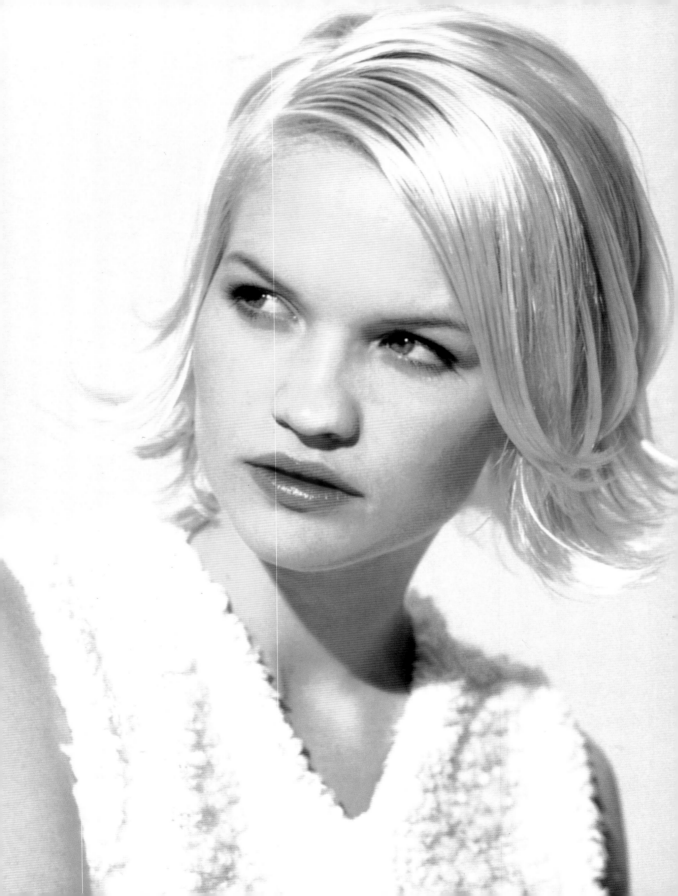

VITAMINS AND SUPPLEMENTS

If we all lived happy, healthy, carefree lives with lots of fresh air, exercise and organically grown foods in an atmosphere that was both pollution- and stress-free we'd probably get all the nutrients we needed from our diet. But this is getting on for the twenty-first century and part of the package is that we live fast, restless lives, often in overcrowded towns and cities. We need all the extra help we can get and if that means taking minerals and vitamins to supplement our diet, so be it. Many vitamins work as antioxidants, helping to protect the system against free radicals that can damage our body cells.

BEST FOR HAIR

- Beta-carotene is converted by the body into vitamin A when required, and it works as an antioxidant, protecting the cells. It helps maintain healthy hair, skin and nails, among other things.
- Vitamin B complex
- Vitamin C
- Omega-3
- Starflower oil
- Selenium
- Zinc

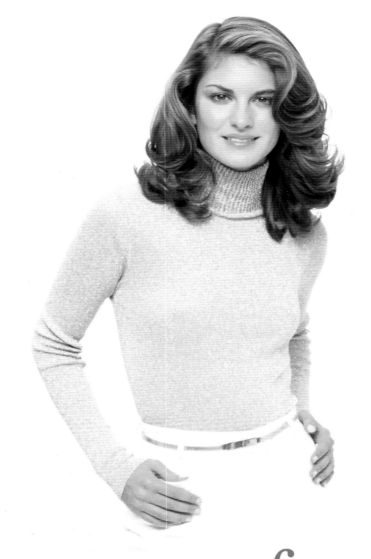

Checklist for Healthy Hair

- If you must have butter rather than a low-fat alternative, use it sparingly.
- Choose semi-skimmed milk rather than the full-fat variety.
- Always buy top-quality oils. Choose ones that name the plant the oil has come from. Avoid generic 'vegetable' oil: it's likely to be made from a mixture of oils and to include additives to prolong its shelf life. Olive oil is considered to be the healthiest option; choose cold-pressed and extra-virgin varieties.
- Eat at least five helpings of fresh fruit and vegetables every day.
- To cook vegetables, steam or stir-fry rather than boil, to keep the nutrients. Or roast or grill them, brushed with a little extra-virgin olive oil.
- Limit cheese and egg intake to a couple of ounces – about 50 grams – of hard cheese a week and no more than four eggs.
- Buy foods as and when you need them. Fresh foods lose too many nutrients while hanging around in your refrigerator. This way you'll also buy fewer processed foods because you'll be resisting the temptation to stock up.
- Eat live yoghurt – our stomach needs certain bacteria to work properly and live yoghurt is a good source of them.
- Complex carbohydrates are sustaining and filling – but watch dressings and toppings. Try baked potatoes without butter but with a little yoghurt and fake caviar. Organically grown spuds should be good enough to eat without any extra help. Avoid creamy sauces with pasta.
- Try to have a vegetarian day each week. You'll be surprised at how easily even a dedicated carnivore can get used to this and how imaginative your meals can be.
- Eat as much raw food as you can, ideally at one meal every day. Again it's surprisingly easy to adjust your diet to this. For breakfast, for instance, have a selection of fruits, or have a large salad for lunch. Otherwise try a huge mound of steamed vegetables for supper, flavoured with fresh herbs or soy sauce.
- Trim excess fat from meat and limit the amount you eat.
- Use fresh herbs and freshly ground black pepper for seasoning and watch your salt intake – try to use salt just in the cooking process and leave it off the table.
- If you really want a bar of chocolate – eat it. But just the one and as the occasional treat. Don't ban your favourite things from your life, because a ban is a punishment and it can't and won't last.
- Be patient – it can take two to three months for dietary changes to show in your hair's condition.
- Don't think about all the things you *can't* eat. Turn the approach around and think about all the items you *can* eat. It's just a change of mindset.

Like any other growing thing, hair needs oxygen. So it's important to get the blood flowing freely around our bodies, taking with it all the oxygen and nutrients that are needed for cell renewal and growth. That's one of the main reasons for taking proper exercise – sure, we all want firm, toned bodies, but getting the necessaries to the bits that need them is of great importance too.

exercise

It takes a lot of pumping to get the blood circulating through our upper torsos, let alone through our shoulders, neck and head. Any encouragement we can give to the coursing of blood through our veins is a good thing.

HAIR EXERCISES

- Breathing always helps! Most of us don't even know how to breathe properly – and it's only by breathing deeply and well that we can get rid of some of the toxins in our bodies as well as helping the oxygen to circulate freely. Most people's breathing is far too shallow and rarely gets past the chest.

- Stand or sit comfortably – you can even lie down for this – and take a really deep breath. You'll know when you're doing it properly because your ribs open up and move to the sides and your stomach expands as your diaphragm moves to accommodate the air. Your shoulders should not be moving but should be relaxed. Now breathe out slowly. Try to take half a dozen deep breaths every so often throughout the day, whenever you have a moment to spare or you think about it. You can do it while standing at the bus stop or while watching TV. Set up an easy rhythm while you do it: breathe in to a count of four, hold for a count of two and breathe out to a count of eight. Proper breathing is the basis of yoga and is also very relaxing. Another exercise is to breathe in through one nostril at a time, holding the other closed, for the same count. Breathe out through the mouth.

- Any cardiovascular exercise is terrific for getting the blood moving. If you can manage twenty minutes' vigorous exercise three or four times a week you'll not only feel better but look better too. However, don't run before you can walk. Indeed, walking itself is great exercise. So if you're not a jogger and haven't run for years – *don't start now*. Simply walk at a brisk pace – no strolling – for twenty to thirty minutes. You should be able to work up a slight sweat and your breathing should increase – that's how you know if you're doing it properly – but slow down if you begin to get out of breath. Get a good rhythm going as you stride out and swing your arms too. If the weather's poor then settle for the treadmill in the gym.

- Cycling is another option and also has a good effect on your thighs.

- Swimming is possibly one of the best overall toning exercises, but the chlorine in pool water and the salt in the sea can play havoc with your hair. To combat chlorine wear a tight-fitting bathing cap or use a product that acts as an invisible bathing cap, such as my Nicky Clarke Sport, the ultimate leave-in conditioner. If you're swimming in the sea try to shampoo or at least rinse out the salt as soon as possible afterwards. If you swim regularly your hair will also benefit from special treatment – a deep nourishing hair mask at least once a week. There's no point wrecking what you are exercising to improve.

- Take up yoga and under proper guidance learn to do a headstand or at least a shoulder stand – both are amazingly good ways of getting blood to the brain and scalp. But only ever do this once you've been taught how to do it properly.

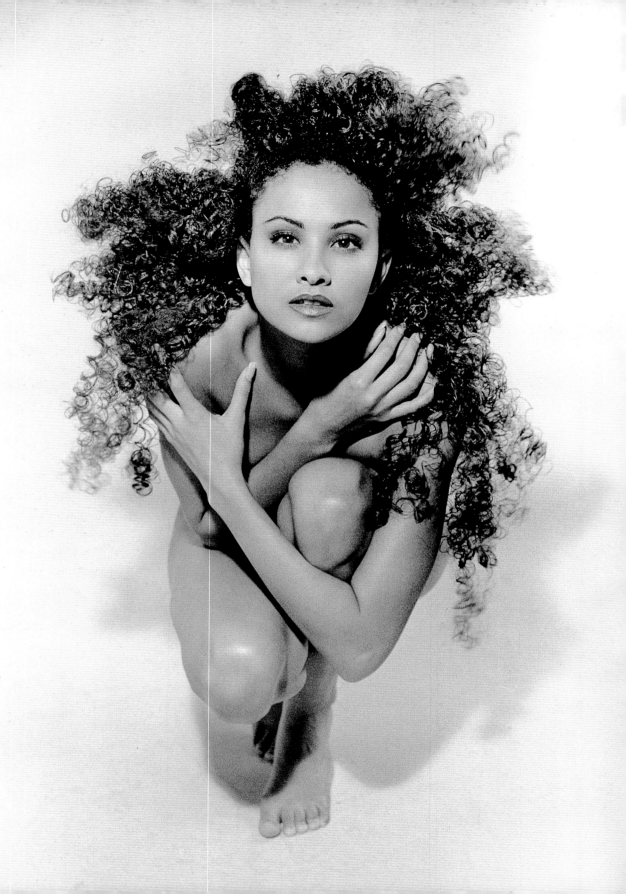

STRESS BUSTING

Some of the hair's greatest enemies are stress, worry and tension. Even the simplest thing, such as the way you sit or stand, can affect your hair's health. If there's too much tension around your neck and shoulders, if you hunch up over a desk or a computer screen, then the supply of blood to these areas and upwards is constricted. That means the oxygen and its accompanying nutrients aren't getting around.

Worry or stress can precipitate anything from bingeing to dandruff. It can make our eyes dull, our skin dry, our hair lank and our bodies listless. It's one of the *bêtes noires* of this century. We live at a rush, work at top speed, take on too many responsibilities, try to pack too much into a day or a week and make unrealistic demands on ourselves, our partners and occasionally our children. When we get to bed we're too exhausted to sleep. We've forgotten the art of relaxation and consequently our systems suffer. A side effect of stress is hair loss, and I don't mean the hundred or so hairs we naturally lose each day. If stress gets too much for us then hair can come out in handfuls. If it's got to that stage it's vital to go to your doctor and if possible a trichologist. But before stress reaches such a peak, teach yourself some relaxation techniques or simply make time in your day for yourself.

Pamper Yourself!

Devoting just five or ten minutes to yourself each day can begin to bring about the most enormous benefits. This may mean a walk in the park and a bit of fresh air, it may mean sitting alone listening to your favourite music, or maybe a wallow in a scented bath at the end of the day. My partner Lesley and I are great believers in aromatherapy and the value of essential oils, which is why we incorporated them into our own hair products. I know that a warm bath with a few drops of lavender or geranium oil can help anybody unwind.

Remember to treat yourself occasionally. There's nothing quite like a reward to make you feel good about yourself and to help relieve the tension. Have a massage on a regular basis. You could even find out if there's a college in your area and get the students to practise on you.

Reflexology is a great soother. If you cannot get to a practitioner then even a good foot massage will help to dissolve tension. Tension often starts at our feet, either because we've been on them all day or because our shoes are too tight.

Learn to massage your own scalp – and you don't have to wait until your next shampoo. Using your fingertips, massage in small circles all over your scalp, starting at the front, working your way around to the sides, then on to the crown and finishing at the back. It stimulates as well as soothes. Do this for two to three minutes, longer if you have time. Then take large chunks of hair and pull upwards away from the scalp – make sure you do this all over the head. Now massage the scalp with the fingertips once more, very vigorously, using short sharp strokes.

For serious stress learn some accepted relaxation technique such as yoga, meditation or self-hypnosis. Each has a way of helping you to calm down. At least practise the breathing exercise above for about five minutes three or four times a day. Or else dance. It's almost impossible to be stressed out while you're dancing. Either do it at home in the privacy of your own kitchen or bedroom, playing your favourite music as loud as you or the neighbours can take it, or join a class and learn to salsa, tango or line dance.

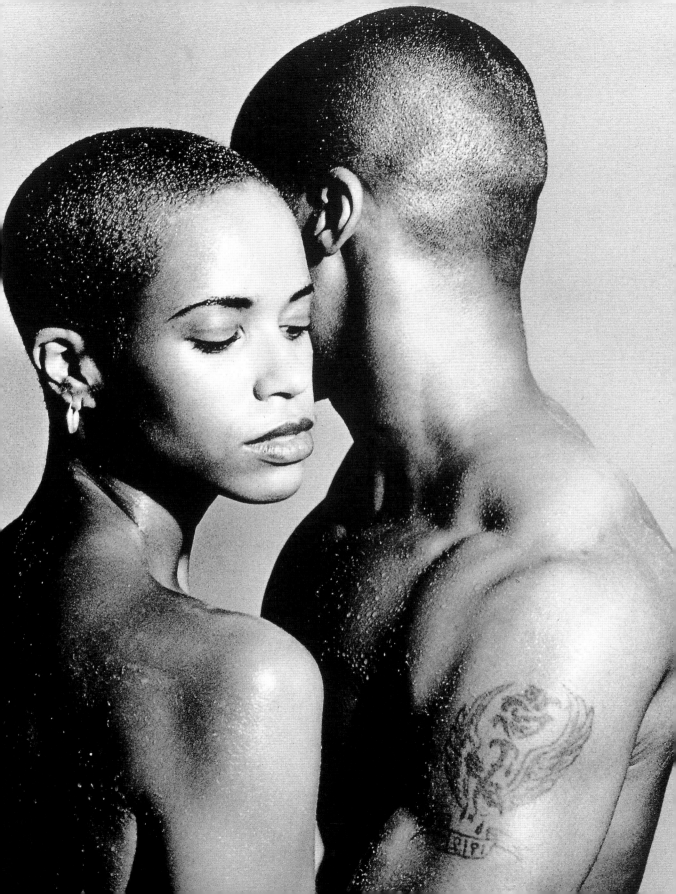

DE-TOX

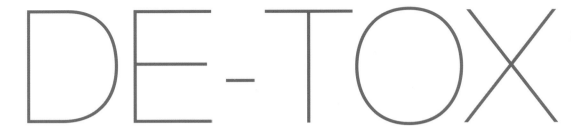

Release those poisonous toxins from your body with a day or two's de-tox diet. You need to take it easy on a de-tox day anyway, and that'll probably help lower your stress in itself. If you've never de-toxed before, begin by doing it for just one day, and make sure you check with your doctor first. Drink only still or purified mineral water and eat only fruit. If you've already invested in a juicer then make your own juices and sip those throughout the day. Most people can take three 8fl oz glasses of fresh juice (that's about 250ml a go) in a day. Here are a few to try:

- orange, grapefruit and lemon, for natural cleansing
- 2 large carrots, 1 orange, 1 stick of celery
- ¼ cucumber, 2 sticks of celery, ¼ melon
- 2 apples, 1 carrot
- 1 apple, 1 kiwi fruit, large slice of melon
- ½ watermelon
- 3 tomatoes, 2 carrots, handful of watercress
- 3 tomatoes, ½ red pepper, 4 spinach leaves
- 1 pear, 1 apple, ½ kiwi fruit
- 1 apple, 6oz (about 175 grams) strawberries

Add herbs such as basil, parsley, ginger or coriander to taste. Soon you'll be able to concoct your own juices, incorporating your favourite ingredients. But do be careful and don't overdo it. Try only one de-tox day at a time. Eventually you'll be able to extend it to two. Throughout the day remember to pamper yourself. Part of the point of this is to relax and suspend normal life for a while. You'll at last have time to do all those beauty treatments you've been promising yourself: a deep hair-conditioning mask, a facial, a manicure and a pedicure.

Be aware of the changing seasons and what they can do to your well-being and your hair. During the winter we stay in overheated houses and places of work, which has a drying effect on our hair. We opt for comforting foods and snacks – though there's no problem here provided you know what's in them and it's good stuff. Cut down on tinned and packet soups, no matter how convenient. It's easy to make your own soups and they taste much better. Keep an eye on your stodge consumption. It's great for quick comfort hits but it can have a sluggish effect on your body. Try not to cut back on visits to the gym or curtail whatever exercise you like doing, even if it's cold and wet outside. You'll feel better after exercise and so will your hair.

During the summer we know that we need to be careful in the sun. We know what its damaging rays can do to our skin and most of us are now well-versed in sunscreen use, but we tend to stop this protection at the hairline. While your hair won't burn and peel it can get severely damaged by exposure to strong UV light. It will dehydrate and its colour will change – colour-treated hair can fade while blonde hair can get overbleached. We need to look after hair in the sun with products that have protective ingredients, such as Hairomatherapy's Frizz Control Shine Serum or Lift Thicken and Shine Styling Spray.

Remember, you don't have to be on holiday to provide your hair with sun-protection. The same rays are working away while you're getting on with your daily life. Also, the best treatment to maintain healthy locks is to shampoo and condition regularly – with perhaps a slightly richer conditioner when you are on holiday.

FINALLY, HERE'S MY HAIR HEALTH BLACKLIST:

POLLUTION
CENTRAL HEATING
CHLORINE
HARD WATER
STRESS
POOR, UNBALANCED DIET
PROCESSED FOODS
SMOKING
TOO MUCH HEAT (FROM HAIR TOOLS)

TRANSFORMATION

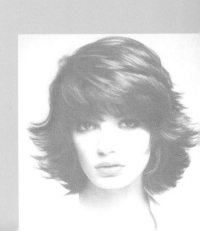

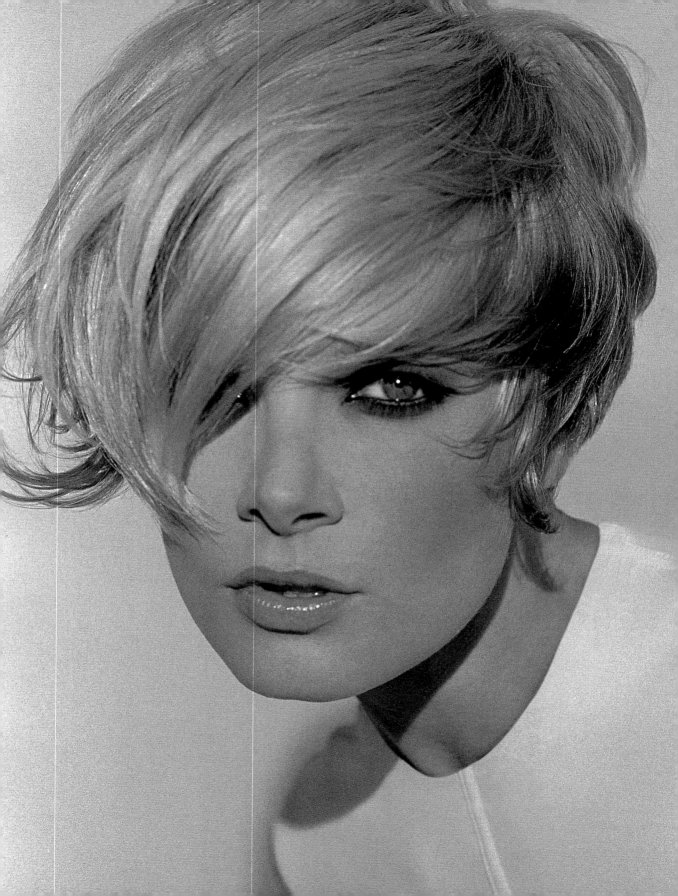

Everybody, no matter what their circumstances or who they are, occasionally wants – and needs – a change. They may be frightened of it, but they still go ahead. It may be a change of job, scene, colour scheme or attitude. Fashion exists thanks to our need for change, but conversely that need for change often has less to do with fashion and more to do with how an individual sees herself, what's being demanded of her and what her emotional needs are at that moment.

One of the simplest and easiest transformations we can make is a change of hairstyle. The lead up to making the decision can be difficult – just as we desire change we're also terrified of it. We might be bored with what we have but we still believe the devil we know is better than the devil we don't – even if the unknown devil is merely a pageboy hairstyle. Our bravado may disappear when we realize we might need to change not only our hairstyle but possibly make-up and accessories to boot. We get used to the way we look. We know how to do it, how to look after it and how to prop it up on a bad day. Often we're so used to it that we don't even see it. But somehow there's a hankering for change. And the only way to do it is to make the decision and jump in.

Some people take time to transform themselves, doing it in stages, while others do it at the drop of a hat. Margaret Thatcher, for instance, took quite some time to develop her style. In the early years of power, both as a minister and then as the prime minister, she had other things to concentrate on, such as her resolute rise to prominence. Once she got the top job and began to realize that how she looked mattered as well as what she did, she attacked the job with her customary zeal. She got somebody to help her with her wardrobe, had her teeth fixed, her voice modulated and began to soften her helmet of hair.

The first thing Mrs T. did was to lighten the colour of her hair: gradually, sensibly and to great effect. The older a woman gets the kinder a lighter shade can be. She also began to soften the helmet effect of her hairstyle – though it was never soft enough for me. I'll never forget the day I went to Downing Street to do her hair for a *Vogue* picture with David Bailey. For the whole thing we were given only thirty minutes: wardrobe, make-up, hair and shoot. Throughout that time three secretaries constantly arrived with briefings, messages and signings for her. The whole thing was mind-boggling, but I loved it. I was a fan, anyway, and whether you agreed with her and what she was doing or not I would defy anybody to say she was not impressive. She was terrific on the day. I had nine minutes to get her hair ready and I spent at least half of that time getting the backcombing out.

Whatever I do and whoever I'm working with I like to introduce a little touch of Nicky Clarke. I thought her hair was too severe and I wanted to make it softer and give it a little more movement without losing any of her stature or dignity. Once I'd got rid of the backcombing I put in strategic bits of volume with a spray and gradually reset it. It must have worked for her because I got a letter a few days later saying how much she liked it and thanking me for the products I'd left for her. As in everything she took a great interest in what people had to say and offer, homing in on what she could use to make her life easier and discarding what she didn't need.

Another client who needs constantly to transform herself from casual to formal without ever losing dignity is Queen Noor of Jordan. She is an extraordinarily sweet and gracious woman with marvellous hair. It's thick and lustrous with a slight wave – quite the best to have for the more formal styles her position often requires. There's very little trouble in anchoring a tiara to this type of hair. Another side to her reflects her more casual American upbringing and comes to the forefront in her travels around Jordan when she spearheads her work on schools, training and conservation. For this she needs what I term 'working hair' – hair that looks good, doesn't require too much upkeep time and doesn't get in the way of concentration, heat or dust. She manages both sides of her life and always looks impeccable.

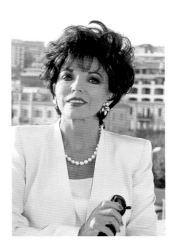

Joan Collins is incredibly impressive and professional. She knows exactly how she likes to look but she's always willing to try something new as well.

On another stellar scale is Joan Collins – also a past mistress of her appearance and in complete control of the effect she creates. More than anything she knows what suits her. Here is a woman who can transform herself four or five times a day. She is clever and canny and over the years has watched, absorbed and learnt from all the professionals around her. She has evolved her own style so completely that she can tell at a glance whether a look, a shade or even an earring is right for her. No photographer, stylist, make-up artist or even hairdresser can do it better than Miss Collins. I once did a cover shoot with her – again with Bailey – for American *Harper's Bazaar*.

She was great fun and very impressive. Everyone knows she wears wigs and she arrived with a selection. Her own hair is fine-textured and she prefers the volume and body, not to mention the changes, that wigs allow her. And, yes, she does appear in public and in movies with her own hair. All those scenes in *Dynasty* showing her with slicked-back short hair? That was her own. Anyway, while we were getting ready for the shoot, and the stylist and make-up artist were going through the wardrobe with her, I began to look at the wigs. I talked her through what she wanted to do with her hair and how she might like to look. With one of those delicious wicked grins she looked at me and said, 'Look, no matter how fantastic you can make my hair look, it will never be as good as any one of these wigs.' Of course we settled for a wig, but styled à la Clarke – soft with a twist!

One person who could not only transform himself overnight but who helped transform an entire generation was Steve Strange. I worked with him a lot because I loved that whole New Romantic movement. It was wild yet incredibly romantic. I was never very good at punk. I found most of it

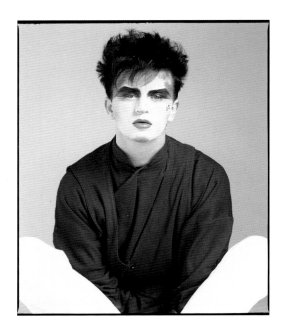

Steve Strange was a

transformation genius –

always looking for

something different,

something new. We had

great times during the

New Romantics era.

ugly and felt alienated by it. But I just loved the entire New Romantics scene. Even the clothes I wore were influenced by it: long boots, frilly shirts, velvet bits. I also loved the hairstyle experimentation that went on: curls, waves, ringlets, extensions, crazy colours of purple, pink and cobalt blue spliced with a little gold. In the Eighties I met all the New Romantics through the Hot Gossip girls and would visit the squat they lived in. I began to do Steve's hair almost from the time we first met and through him I met and worked with Adam Ant and Billy Idol. Every night these guys would try a different look or a different style: no wonder they captured everyone's imagination. Except I suppose that in the end the real world intrudes and somehow you need to get back to normal life, although you take a lot of the lessons you learned with you. This again underlines my philosophy of wearable styles that are never dull or ordinary. A mix of the radical with the mainstream.

It is extraordinary just what a radical change can bring about. Possibly my most famous client is the Duchess of York and I was both responsible for and a supporter of one of the most radical transformations she's ever had. But it didn't start out that way. The whole thing was quite spontaneous. I'd been doing her hair for about eighteen months when it happened. The occasion was another *Tatler* cover shoot, again with Terry O'Neill. The Duchess had recently given birth to Princess Eugenie and like many women her hair post-pregnancy was dull, lifeless and limp. She was used to none of these things. Usually she has masses of vibrant, healthy hair. It was the only time I ever thought of suggesting a colour rinse to bring some oomph back into her natural red – but I didn't. Instead I began to think around the problem.

During most cover sessions we try three or
four different shots to give both the editor
and art director a choice. Then, if there's
time, we'll do a couple more fashion-type
pictures with possibly just a change of dress
or pose. In the first picture from this session
the Duchess's hair was long, but it needed a
lot of work to bring out its natural vitality
and vibrancy, particularly under the strong
studio lights and the harsh white
background. She and I were looking at a
couple of the Polaroids (a photographer
always takes these first to check the lights
and outline), when I suggested that her hair
needed to be shorter to get some movement
and shape back into it. And that's how it
started. 'I suppose you're just dying to cut
it,' she said to me, and oddly enough I wasn't
desperate to cut it, but somehow we ended
up with the most spectacular bob – which
she loved, and no matter what the
newspapers said afterwards so did Prince
Andrew.

Along with this totally different hairstyle she
needed a new style of dressing. I'd been
steering her away from her old, rather fussy
style ever since I'd started to do her hair.
When she first asked me to look after her
hair she'd been going through a phase of
fussy accessories. Flowers, combs, pins, slides
and jokey bits like helicopters all found their
way onto her red curls. I'd been gradually
eliminating them and also styling her hair in
a much simpler fashion. As we got to know
each other she began to trust my judgement
and asked me for advice more and more
about what she should wear for which
occasion. It began with hats and tiaras, but
these needed to match what she was wearing.

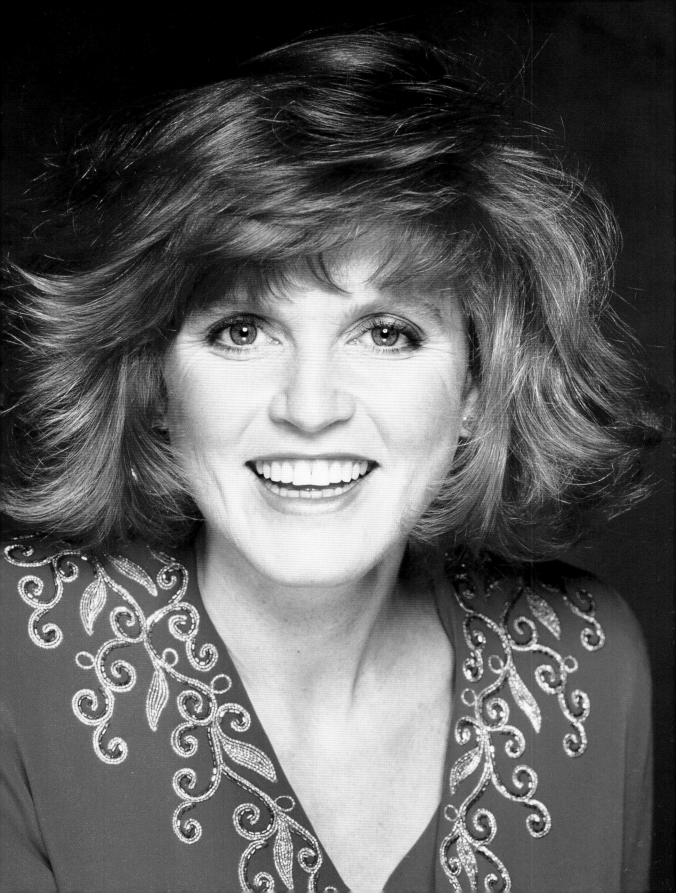

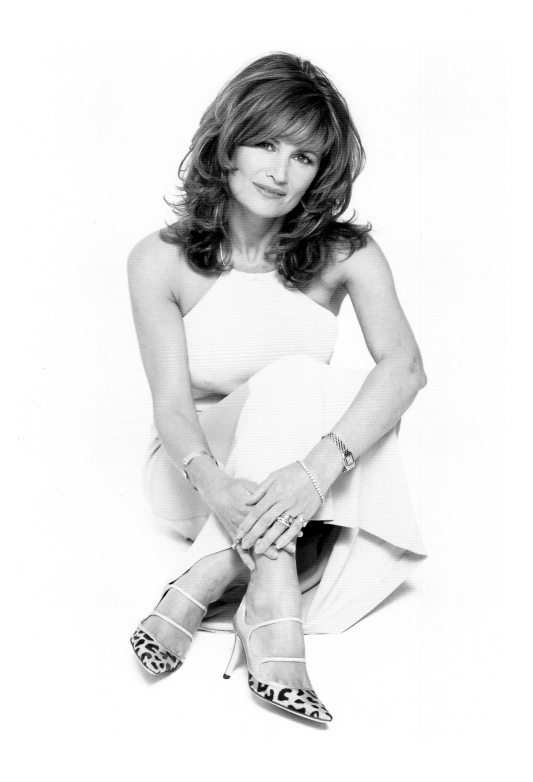

My wife Lesley has fantastic style and great taste. She would often help on shoots: she was a fashion designer before we started the business. She helped restyle the Duchess of York.

At the Palace she'd ask me to look in the wardrobe and see what would be right for whatever engagement she had.

Gradually she began to discard some of the fluffier and fussier jobs. And this was where my wife, Lesley, came into her own. Before Lesley and I began to work together she'd been a fashion designer. She has impeccable taste. If I was with the Duchess and she had a problem about what to wear, I'd call Lesley and give her the problem to solve. Gradually Lesley began to come to the Palace with me and helped reorganize the Duchess's wardrobe. She introduced her to a completely different set of designers: those who produce very classic, simple clothes exquisitely made from gorgeous fabrics. People like Anoushka Hempel and Anthony Price. All those amazingly simple rich velvet dresses in purple, dark green and chocolate brown that the Duchess was photographed wearing were from that period. This whole transformation stemmed from a different hairstyle.

While a change from long to short hair can be dramatic, nothing has quite the impact of a change of colour. Nobody knows this better than top model Linda Evangelista who has, over the last ten years, been every colour you can think of and often two or three shades at one time. But then she has the panache to carry it off, as well as the good fortune to have looks that any colour will suit. She also has the savvy to change her make-up and accessories along the way. What looks good on a sunkissed blonde doesn't have the same effect on a sultry brunette or a sock-'em-in-the-teeth redhead.

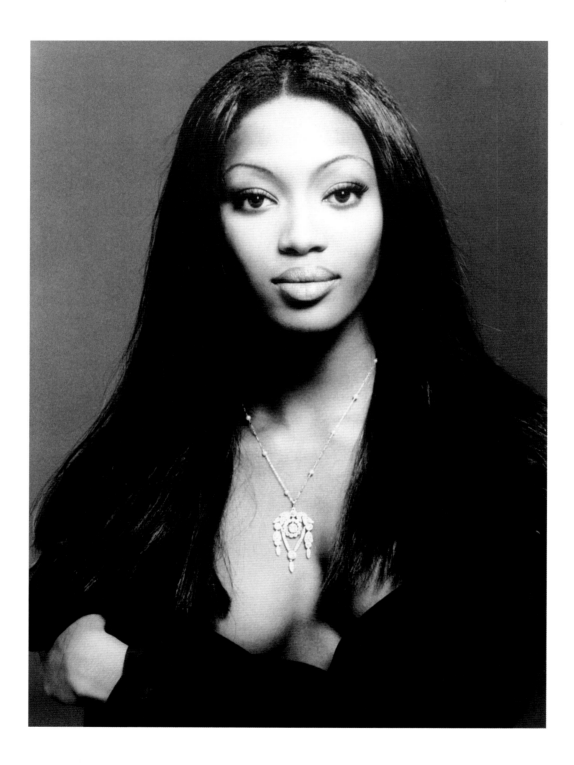

Top models know only too well what a serious change of colour can do for them. Nadia Auerman was just another long, lean body until she went platinum blonde and turned into an icon of the late Eighties, while Karen Elson was just another unusual-looking young hopeful until photographer Steven Meisel decreed that she should change to a strong red and shave off her eyebrows to boot.

But whatever transformation you are after you must realize one thing: the style you opt for in the end *must* have flexibility. You'll feel much more comfortable knowing that it's versatile and that you can change the look by styling it a different way, by making it curlier, straighter or by adding accessories. Even the Rachel style, as Jennifer Aniston's is called, can be worn in several different ways: just watch any half-hour of *Friends* and you'll see how many permutations it has. I'm convinced that's one of the reasons for its popularity – it's a style that's simple and yet never appears boring. And nobody's ever remarked that here are people allegedly with no money who have some of the most desirable styles on the planet. If the style you choose is versatile you won't regret it and you'll rarely be bored.

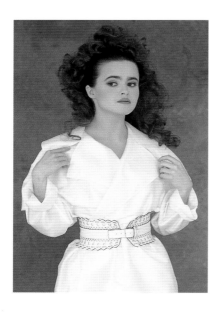

Helena Bonham-Carter has naturally luxuriant, wavy hair. However, she often uses wigs and pieces for period movie roles.

One simple way to transform hair is with a hairpiece. People sometimes look at me as if I've gone mad when I suggest they use one and even more so if I suggest they take one away on holiday with them. Many actresses and models spend their lives surrounded by wigs and hairpieces and nobody thinks they're crazy. Movie stars whose hair we admire and want to copy often wear wigs or pieces in films. Even Helena Bonham-Carter in the middle of her costume dramas and in spite of her own luxuriant locks was enmeshed in hairpieces. Most of the weird and wonderful hairstyles you see at catwalk fashion shows are done with wigs – I know because we do quite a lot of them, most recently Alexander McQueen's. What's more, they don't have to cost a fortune. If you want to look natural then make sure they match your own hair colour. And these days they are so well put together you need never see the join.

I have a number of clients who take up to three hair pieces away on holiday with them – but even taking one makes a lot of sense, particularly if you have curly or frizzy hair prone to the effects of humidity. The added advantage of a hair piece on holiday is that it allows you to look glam when you've no time to get ready, or when the electricity in your hotel or villa is playing up and your styling brush or dryer won't work. At times like these you'll be grateful for that hairpiece. Or think of it as protection. Your own hair can be scraped back with a sunscreen, conditioner or gel and the fake piece can take most of the sun's damaging rays.

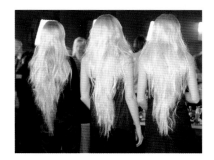

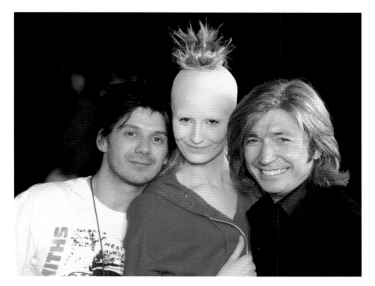

*With Erin O'Connor and
Guido, who leads my
International Fashion Team
– creating the styles for major
catwalk shows – here behind the
scenes at Alexander McQueen.*

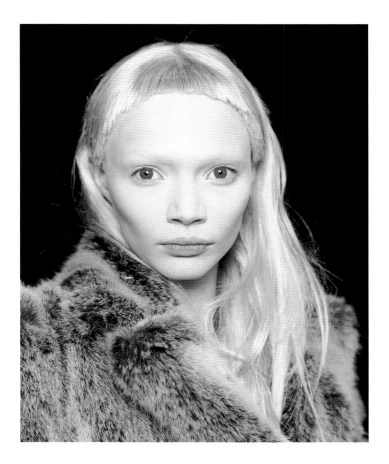

Jodie Kidd at the same show.

VERSACEJ
ILSANDER
RMcQUEE
NCALVINK
LEINLOUI
SVUITTON
GIVENCHY

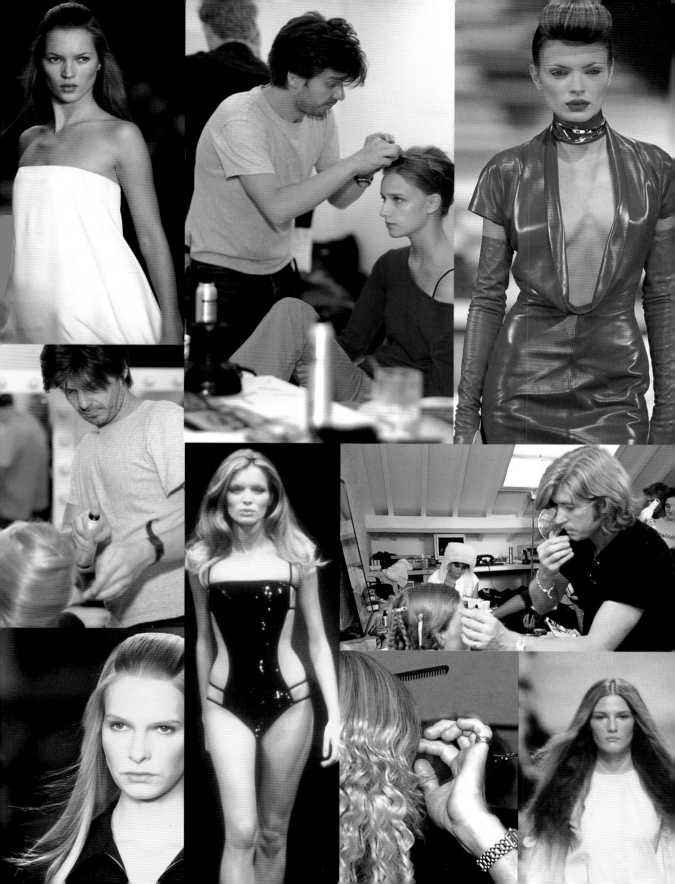

WIG POWER

The great thing about wigs and hairpieces today is that there are so many different types. There are those made from real hair, which are put onto machine-made bases and cost anywhere between £30 and £300. Then there are the synthetics, which these days are very good – and they are cheaper (£30 to £200), lighter and more accessible. Each has its advantages. It's down to you to decide which you feel best with and which you can afford. However, what is certain is that more and more people are using them, and not just for photographic shoots and runway shows, where they come into their own for continuity of look and for speed. Lots of people are putting them on for a special party or a fun night out, or just to boost their own hair into that instant babe look.

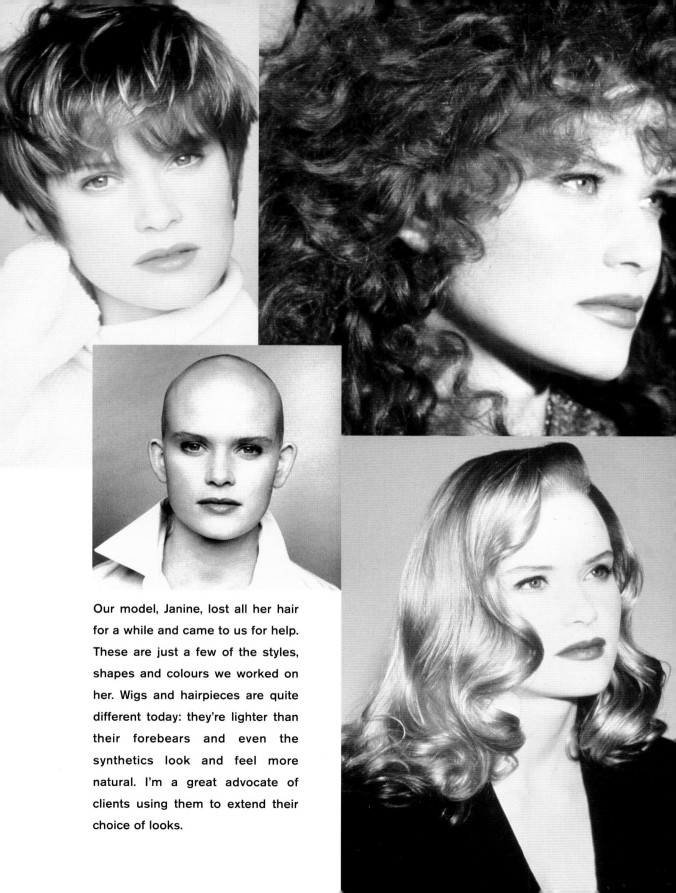

Our model, Janine, lost all her hair for a while and came to us for help. These are just a few of the styles, shapes and colours we worked on her. Wigs and hairpieces are quite different today: they're lighter than their forebears and even the synthetics look and feel more natural. I'm a great advocate of clients using them to extend their choice of looks.

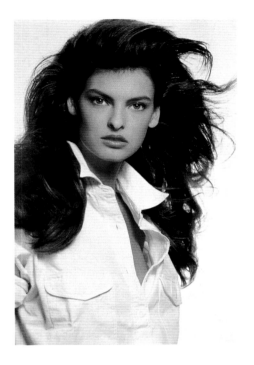

Supermodel Linda Evangelista, famous for her many hair changes, here with a hairpiece for a Vogue *shoot.*

The most usual pieces are the three-quarter-head piece and the ponytail piece. Of three-quarter-head pieces, some, particularly the synthetic variety, now come on toothed alice bands which hold to the head really well. Otherwise it's best to pin-curl the back of the hair or backcomb it so the piece has something to latch on to. Flat silky hair is not an ideal fixing point. Ponytail pieces are easy and becoming popular because the ponytail is turning into the modern-day classic long hairstyle. It's almost the chignon for the late twentieth century.

The best wigs for my purposes are those made from fine European-type hair. Most of them are made by John Clifton, whose wigs are shown on page 117. John has invented a base that's light and thin, as well as a unique knotting technique which means the wigs look incredibly natural and can be parted any way.

Extensions, which immediately give you longer thicker hair, can be made from either real hair or synthetics. Again, each has its advantages: one is less expensive, and the other is more natural in feel, but new developments and processes are being introduced all the time. Extensions are very popular and growing more so. They began with the Afro market and then took off with Boy George and the dreads. One of their disadvantages is that the wearer very quickly gets used to having one and when the extension is taken out sometimes thinks that their own hair has been damaged. Mostly it hasn't – it's just that their own hair feels finer by comparison.

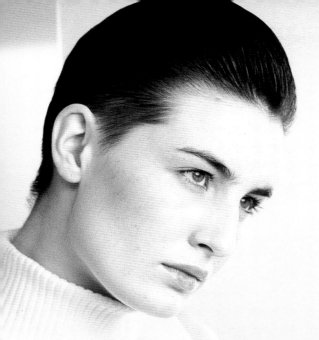

ERIN O'CONNOR

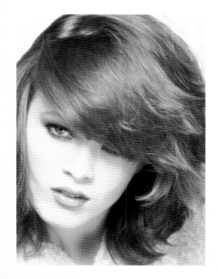

KAREN ELSON

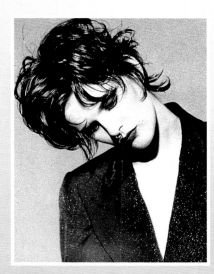

STELLA TENNANT

SORRY, KARL, WE GOT THERE FIRST!

Top designer Karl Lagerfeld has a habit of choosing stunning British models to act as his 'muse' for the look of the top Paris fashion house, Chanel. These girls are guaranteed massive international recognition and, usually, lucrative advertising contracts. It's funny that, over the years at Nicky Clarke, we have always managed to catch exactly the same models early in their careers. You might say BC — Before Chanel!

CHOOSING YOUR TRANSFORMER

Sometimes a hairdresser gets credited with magical powers and properties that are way beyond his experience. A hairdresser cannot change your life but he can allow you to, by helping you to achieve the looks and get the confidence you need. Hairdressers have the knowledge, experience, a facility to style and an interest in making someone look their best and achieve their potential. I get branded as the man with the magic scissors and the million-dollar touch, but that's because I've devised my own way of dealing with hair over twenty years. I've managed to create my own method of seeing and understanding the potential each person has, and making it happen.

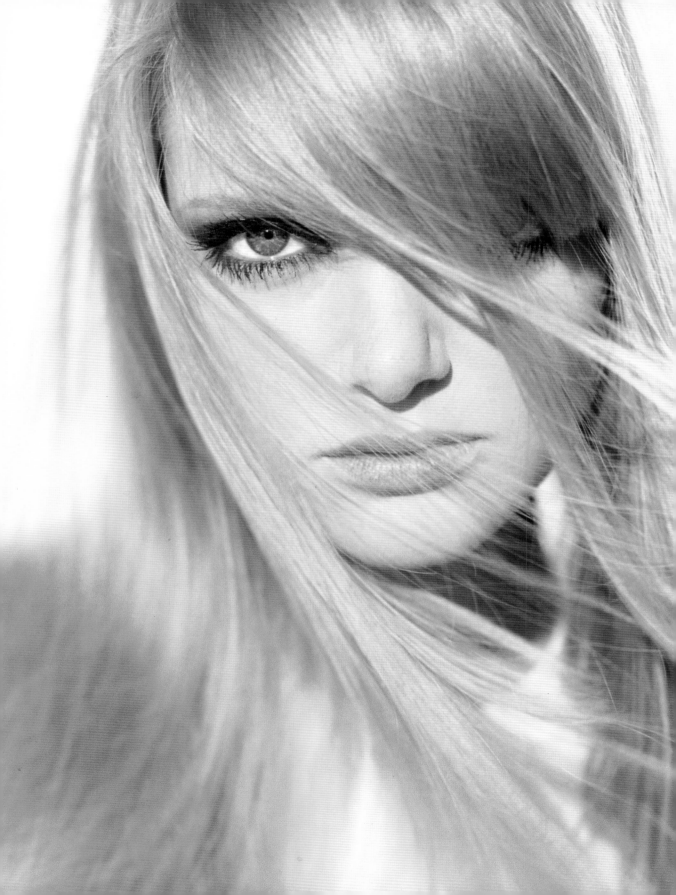

■ Step One: Still the best way of finding a hairdresser is by word of mouth. Ask your friends and the people you work with who they rate. If you ever see someone whose hairstyle you like in the street, a shop, a club or at work, *ask* them where they had it done. I know it sounds very American to go up and tell somebody how much you like their hair – but Americans get things done, and most people are flattered if you compliment them and more than delighted to tell you which salon was responsible.

■ Step Two: Once you have established which hairdresser it is to be, talk to him or her at length. Book yourself in for a consultation. Occasionally a hairdresser who knows he's good feels he doesn't need to offer a consultation before someone makes up their mind about booking in for a restyling, but that doesn't happen often. Neither I nor my staff have ever felt that way. We always find time to talk to a potential client, even if it's only for five or ten minutes. We don't even ask that they book in for a consultation. Anyone can come along and someone will always see them for a few minutes. It gives the client a chance to weigh up what sort of person you are and whether you could get along together, and also what the salon and its atmosphere are like.

■ Step Three: If a consultation is not on offer but you still want to visit that salon or person, then simply book in for a blow-dry. You may find resistance from a prima donna hairdresser who feels that he or she cannot work with somebody else's cut. I find that attitude arrogant. It's on a par with a stylist who proceeds to rubbish the style you were given by your last hairdresser. However, only you the client can decide whether this behaviour is acceptable or not. And indeed some people welcome that sort of attitude because they feel that's what they are paying for – to be told what to do. Added to which you may like the salon and its atmosphere and you may want the person to do your hair because they've been highly recommended. It's horses for courses.

Personally, I think it's bad manners to rubbish somebody else's work, but sometimes you need to point out what is wrong in order to rectify it. If you think you've got a bit of a turkey of a style then you'll know if you've found the right person to rectify it because he or she will be honest with you, tell you what can be done with it in the immediate future and

promise that if you both stick with the remedy until the change is fully achieved you'll look a great deal better and feel happier. Most people are grateful for that sort of honesty from a hairdresser: it doesn't offer miracles but it promises gradual improvement. That in many cases is the beginning of a lifelong, trusting relationship.

■ Step Four: Try not to rush things. Give yourself time to get to know your new hairdresser, and give him or her a chance to find out about your hair, how you like to look and how much time you're prepared to spend looking after it. If you're not satisfied with the initial result tell your hairdresser and explain what exactly you don't like – give him or her a chance to rectify it. Remember that until about an hour ago you were complete strangers to each other.

■ Step Five: Once you've discussed what style you want and have agreed with the stylist (and this may not be on the first visit), then let him (or her) get on with the job. He has the professional experience, you've chosen him for it, and you have to let him get on with it. You *cannot* change your mind halfway through, because it not only invalidates the discussions you've had up till then and the idea that you've both come up with, it also undermines his ability as well as his confidence.

The art of a good hairdresser is to know what sort of client he's dealing with. If she's fashion-conscious, then it's important to allow her to keep abreast of trends. But even if she's not so fashion-conscious, it doesn't mean she doesn't want to move with the times. A good hairdresser knows this, and should be able constantly to update a style or look. Often it's no more than a tweak here or a flick there, or maybe the introduction of a fringe.

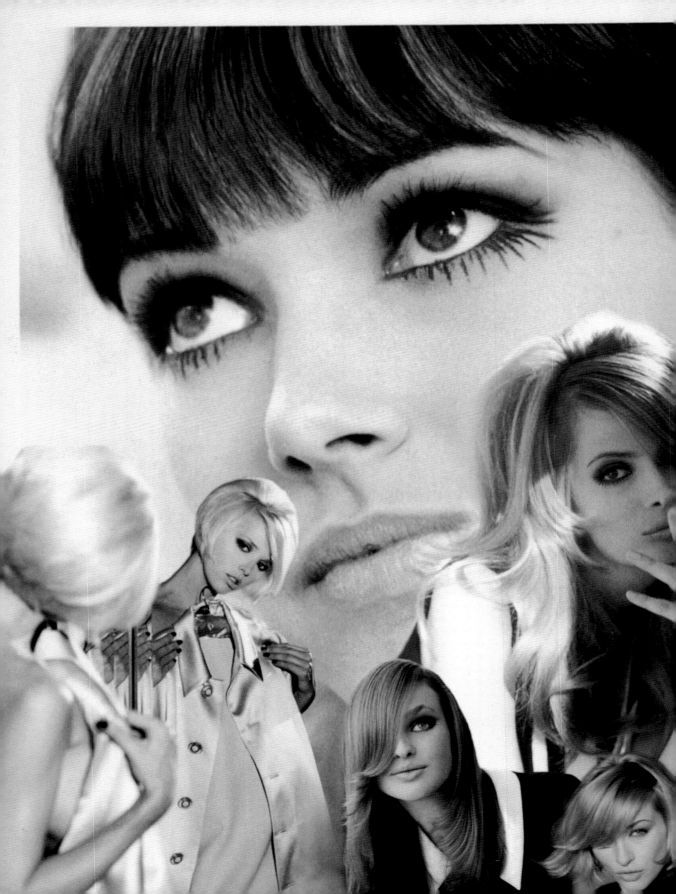

Time for a Change?

Once you have found a hairdresser whose work you like and whose opinions you trust it's usually a relationship for life. But every so often a client feels a stylist has lost interest in her hair. If this happens to you, you need to communicate your fears and worries to your stylist. It may be as simple as that, or it may be a matter of asking someone else to do your hair for a while. If and when you return to your original stylist, it's his or her responsibility to let your absence pass unnoticed.

It's happened to me on a few occasions, but when people have returned, which they generally do after a few weeks, I've been scrupulous not to refer to it. I never say anything about their absences because I don't want to put any client in the position of having to justify their choices.

Some clients are open about such a situation – and that's nice and grown-up. They've come back and told the truth – it was nothing personal but they just fancied a change. I make sure to show them how happy I am that they've come back, but I also point out that it's their money and it's entirely up to them who they choose to spend it with. The emotional drain of finding another stylist and building up a new relationship is probably too much for a lot of people. But it's the job of the hairdresser to make the client feel comfortable no matter what she chooses to do.

There are times when a client finds a new hairdresser they think is better than the previous one and more sensitive to their needs. Maybe the client prefers the way number-two stylist does her hair and decides to stick with him. If this happens to you as a hairdresser there's nothing you should do about it – the customer chooses. But it's good manners as well as friendly to say hello when you see your former client and comment on how fabulous her hair is looking. It's important that the hairdresser keeps such a relationship going and never closes the door.

But if a relationship has hit rock bottom and trust has been broken, there's only one thing to do – find a new stylist. Familiarity can breed complacency and both client and hairdresser are aware of this. Most women know when their hair is going wrong. That's the time to discuss it with your current hairdresser – if you want to. If your hairdresser is being non-communicative and a touch arrogant and you're still unhappy, then perhaps it really is time to move. It's your hair, and your needs must be met.

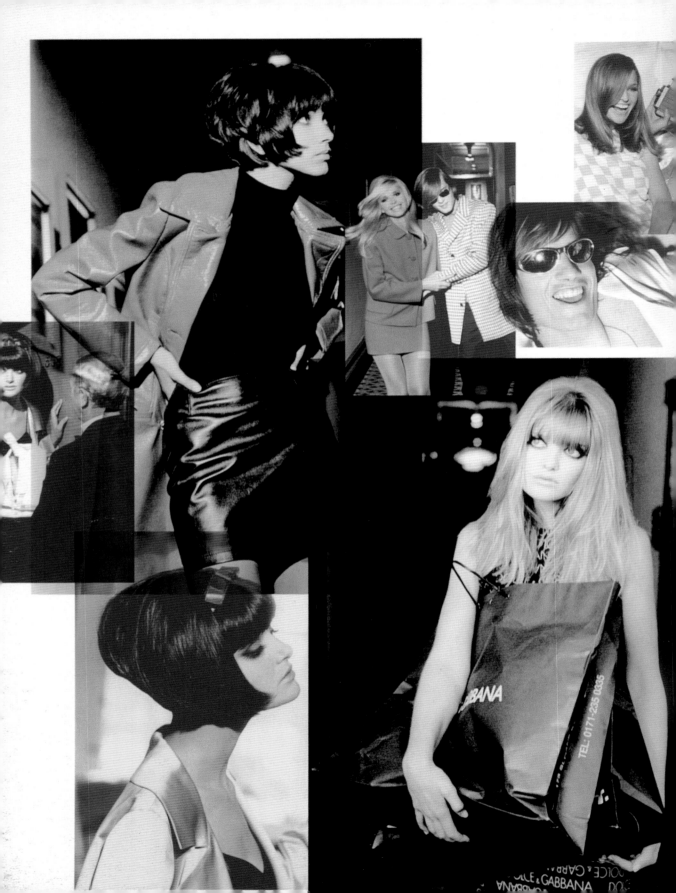

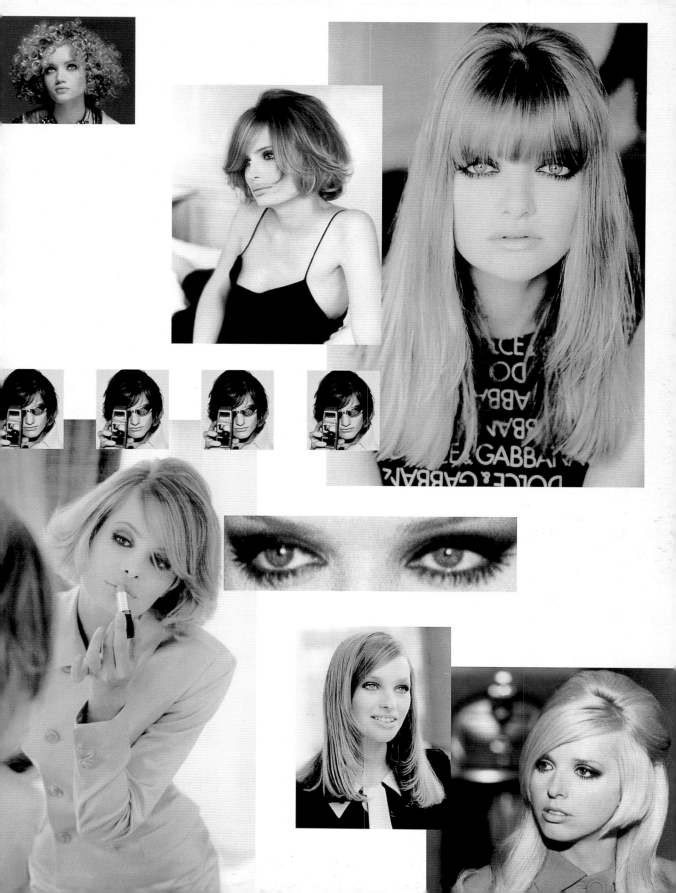

ARE YOU A RADICAL OR A CONSERVATIVE?

Some women (and a lot of men, for different reasons) find a look and stick with it for most of their lives. There are two sorts of people here. One sort are those who are stuck in a time warp and haven't changed their look for years. Believe me, there are any number of these. Nothing's more ageing than a look that's past its prime and what's sad is that it's often a look that was terrific at first – but the wearer has changed in the meantime and the look hasn't evolved.

The biggest culprit is the leftover from the bubble perm that turned into the wash-and-wear perm. You can still see it on thousands of people, stuck somewhere in the mid-Seventies, in towns and cities throughout the country. Its attraction was understandable right from the beginning. Before then perms had meant careful setting

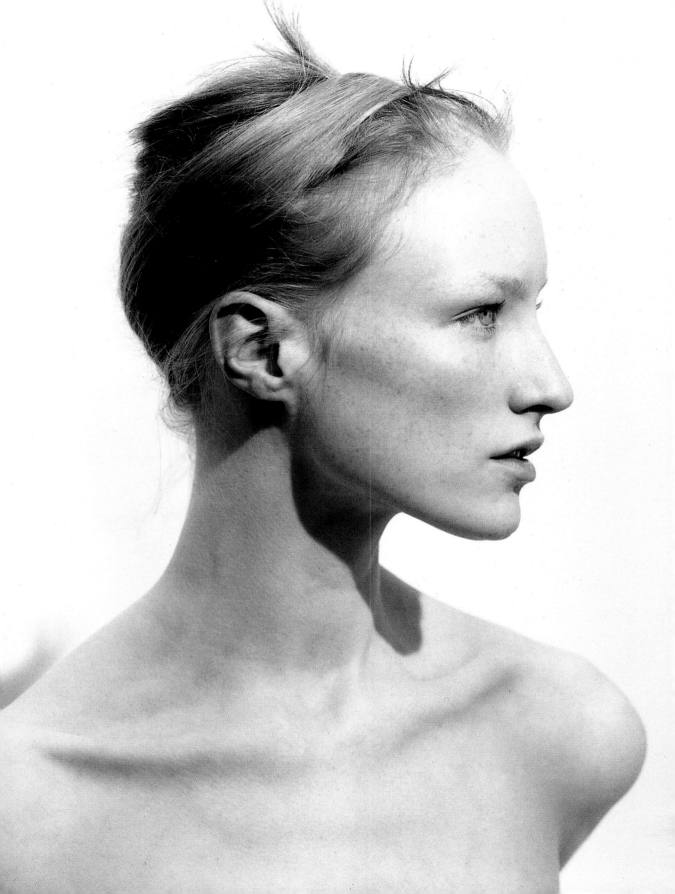

with proper rollers and lotions and a lot of effort so they did not degenerate into a frizz. So when this softer approach arrived – on everybody from Barbra Streisand to Martin Shaw – and all you had to do was shampoo and pat the excess moisture out of it with a towel, it seemed like the answer to life. The easiest hairstyle ever invented, and a godsend to people with fine, limp hair. But, like everything else, it evolved – the perm evolved. A new version of it arrived which imparted *body* rather than *curl* and was to make an even greater contribution to hairstyles. But people had got used to the ease of the wash 'n' wear. They didn't want to change. They didn't realize that all around them things were changing: fashion, make-up, shades, colours. Occasionally they would shift to a newer skirt length or go from colour on the face to neutrals, but the old bubble curls stayed the same. Changing a lipstick doesn't modernize something that's inherently out of date.

> It didn't even have to be a major change – perhaps a shorter cut, a looser perm or using different products with modern blow-drying techniques. *Coronation Street*'s Deirdre Barlow has an awful lot to answer for because she kept the whole thing going during the Eighties! Glenn Close gave it a new twist in *Fatal Attraction* – shorter and looser – but her character must have put the frighteners on people because they didn't stream into the hairdresser's demanding a *Fatal* perm.

Then there's the woman who knows what suits her and stays within those guidelines without ever looking out of date. This is the woman who keeps an eye on changing trends but is also aware of how her face, body and attitude changes, and knows how to adapt trends to suit her. Bryan Ferry's wife, Lucy, is one such woman. Even though she changes her looks, she still maintains that sleek edge, whether it is a sharper style or a softer one, whether it is lighter or darker. Throughout she has retained her own definite look. One time it may have had a heavier fringe, then a lighter version, then none at all – she has constantly kept abreast of what's happening. And her husband is exactly the same – from those early forehead flicks to today's gentler version, he still looks great and as fashionable as next season's clothes.

Then there are the women who change their hairstyle and colour all the time. That's mostly because they are serious followers of fashion or have a low boredom threshold. Sometimes it's lack of confidence, but eight times out of ten it's to stay in fashion.

For the majority of people the sensible road to take is to find your own style, the one you feel comfortable with and the one that gives you confidence in your own looks, and stick to it. But also try to recognize when it's time to adapt – and this is where your stylist comes in. If you've got the right one – and I still believe there are many more good hairdressers than bad ones out there – he or she will make suggestions when it's time to change. It may be just a little shift to begin with, but gradually you might go for more radical change. Try not to panic. Remember: it's in your hairdresser's interest to keep you looking your very best.

Also, as we get older our face shape changes – gravity gets in on the act – and skin tones can get sallow or dull, so it makes sense that hair shape, shade and occasionally colour should try to compensate for these changes. It may be that you need only an infinitesimal shift in style but that shift will keep you looking fresh rather than jaded.

There'll always be the extremes such as punk, gothic, the New Romantics and grunge, and while they appeal mostly to a minority – the young and the ultra fashionable – they do leave a lasting legacy. Punk, for instance, became more mainstream when its gravity-defying elements met the heads of well-groomed women, while the more outrageous colours it sported – pink, purple and bright blue – can now, with the advent of hair mascara, be streaked on for a special event. The asymmetric cuts of the Romantics can be seen in various forms, from those currently worn on the catwalks of the world to one of the currently most copied styles, that worn by Natalie Imbruglia – a mixture of romanticism and grunge.

THE RADICALS
AMONG MY FAVOURITES ARE LINDA EVANGELISTA, NICK RHODES, DEMI MOORE, MEG RYAN, JOHN GALLIANO, MADONNA AND DAVID BOWIE.

THE CONSERVATIVES
TOP OF THE BUNCH ARE MARIA SHRIVER, CHRISTY TURLINGTON, CLAUDIA SCHIFFER, ELIZABETH HURLEY, BRYAN FERRY, PATSY KENSIT, JEMIMA KHAN AND HRH QUEEN NOOR OF JORDAN.

Fringe Benefits

■ An easy, quick and not at all radical way to give any style a lightning transformation is with a fringe. Whatever style of fringe you opt for – short, long, thick, spiky, soft or hard, a fringe invariably makes you look younger, softer, sexier.

■ You need to change and adapt a fringe to reflect changes in style and age. A fringe that's too heavy adds to the effect of gravity so you need to lighten and soften it as you get older. It's extraordinary how many different types of fringe there are: from the Cleopatra block to the Jemima Khan wisp and the Karen Elson high cut.

■ Fringes are flattering and flirtatious. In one instant they draw attention to the eyes, which they highlight and emphasize, at the same time as giving you something to hide behind to impart an air of mystery. Look at how Elizabeth Taylor used her Cleopatra fringe to draw attention to her amazing eyes, while Liam Gallagher uses his to look dangerously sexy.

■ Most young people can take a thick heavy fringe. Look at the Beatles, but see too how Paul McCartney has softened his fringe over the years.

■ Amanda Pays, another long-standing client, has adopted a much wispier version as the years have gone by. When I cut Selina Scott's hair very short I gave her that heavy fringe to add sophistication to her short style, and then when she began to grow it we made it lighter.

■ For really strong, perfectly shaped faces, such as those of Julie Ann Rhodes and Yasmin Le Bon, a fringe gives a softer appeal and makes them look more approachable.

■ A light fringe, such as the one worn by the Duchess of York, suits most people and most styles. I've styled similar ones for clients such as Sinead Cusack and Claudia Schiffer. The styles may be as chalk and cheese but the fringe works fantastically well with both.

■ It's amazing how easily you can change an image just by cutting a fringe. Elaine Paige wanted to look funkier so I gave her a spiky version – she loved it, and the bonus was that it made her look younger too.

■ I made Isabella Rossellini's a very short, very *parisienne* fringe – one that takes a lot of confidence to carry off. It added to the sophistication of her look. We had great fun working on a session, which included film and photographic work, as well as the cover of *Marie Claire* – to think that when I was first asked to do it I nearly refused because it was to take so many days out of the salon! A similar type of fringe was recently sported by model Karen Elson but because her features are much bigger than Rossellini's the fringe looks distinctive and funky on her.

■ The great thing about a fringe is that you can curl it, wave it, grow it, brush it to one side or slick it back for a different look. That's why fringes are such great favourites with everybody. The easiest one is the wispy.

■ The fringe is a great disguiser too. It can disguise thinning hair at the front and sides, and it can cover up a high, low or uneven hairline.

■ Best of all, a fringe can make anyone look younger. Oddly enough, you can run into problems with its youth-bestowing potential. My daughter, Tellisa, for instance, does not want a fringe and will not have one – for what self-respecting nine-year-old wants to look like a six-year-old?

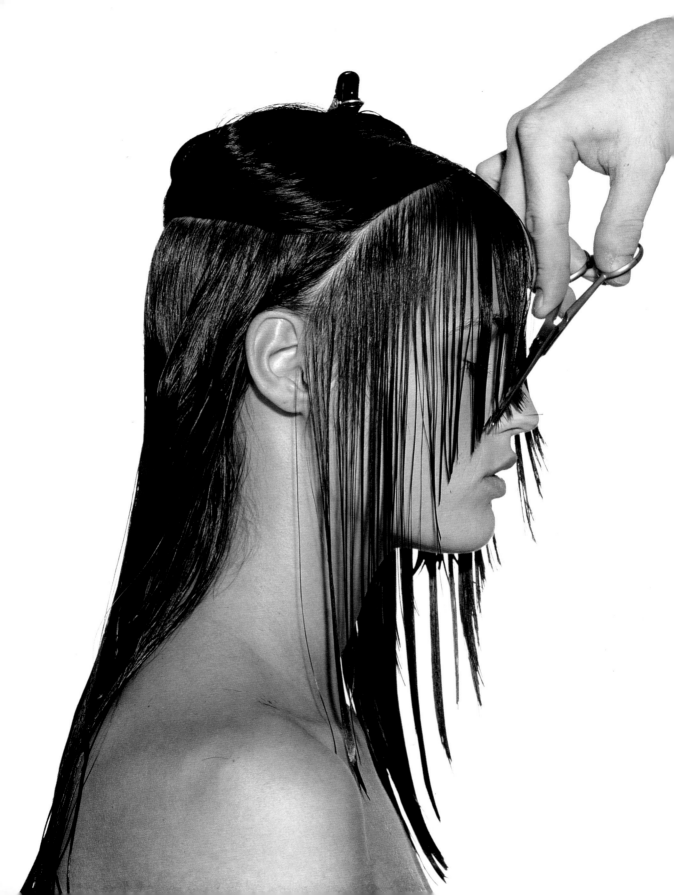

BIG MISTAKE?

IF, AFTER ALL YOUR TIME AND EFFORT,

YOU ARE UNSURE ABOUT YOUR TRANSFORMATION,

REMEMBER THESE THREE THINGS:

1.

Even though you may not like it at first or it may come as a bit of a shock, it may just be a style that needs a little getting used to. It may be a matter of time, or a matter of experimenting with the way you dry it and the products you use.

2.

If you still don't feel right, remember the great thing about hair – it grows. In the meantime, you can change its texture or its colour either permanently or temporarily.

3.

Embrace it and remind yourself that a good new hairstyle is like a facelift without the surgery. That's no exaggeration. It's both costly and painful to change the shape of your face or any of its features but a flick here, a sweep back there or a shorter cut at the nape can give the illusion of much greater change *and* can be done in an hour or two.

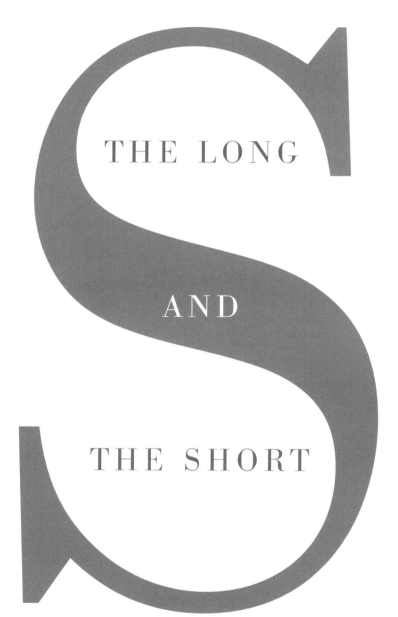

THE LONG

AND

THE SHORT

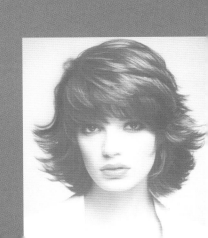

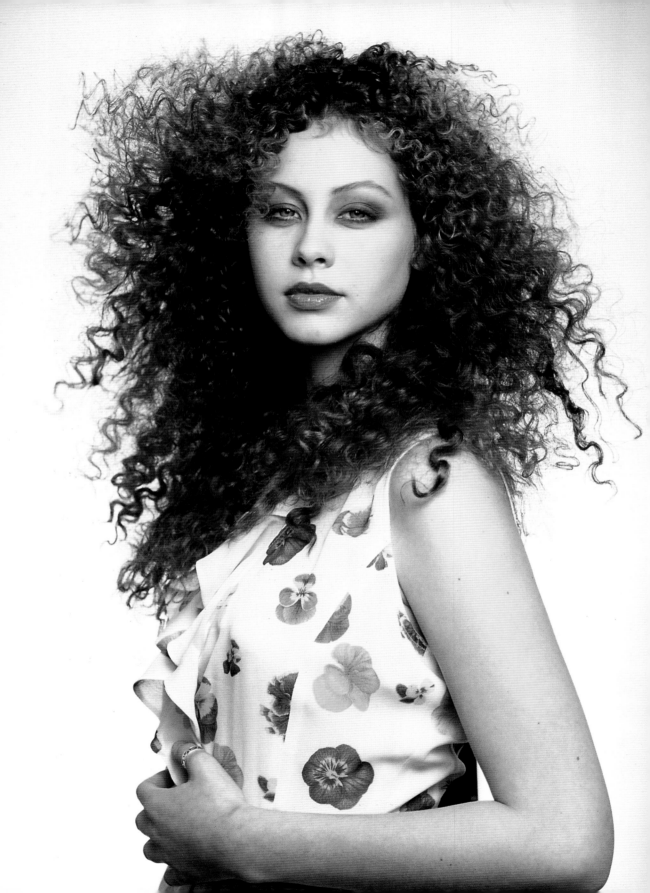

long

I'm better known now for the short hairstyles I've created, but in the early part of my career I was mostly recognized for long styles. Particularly in the early Eighties, when the fashion was for the New Romantics, and even before that, when I was evolving new styles for the dance group Hot Gossip, I spent most of my creative time working with long hair. Long hair demands commitment and a completely different approach from both stylist and wearer. Some stylists are terrific at coping with long hair and others quite the opposite.

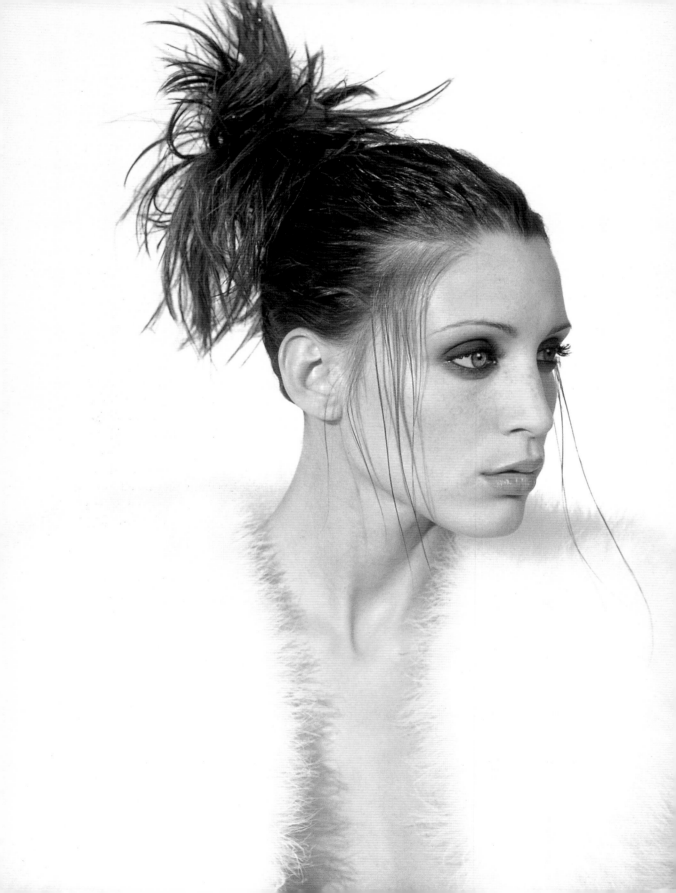

When you start in hairdressing, one of the early parts of your training is how to cut hair – even the longest varieties need trimming. When I began, I was so nervous that I used to watch for the girls coming in on training night who had long hair. I'd make a beeline for them, confident that all they'd want was a slight trim. I could do that easily. But one night I got it wrong. I'd picked one such girl and she told me she wanted the whole lot off and layered. I panicked and hid in the bathroom for three hours. Fortunately, that was the only time I lost my nerve. Once I'd got through this barrier, things began to improve. Learning to cope with, cut or style hair is like learning anything else – to begin with you're full of enthusiasm, then you go through a phase of knowing all the moves but not understanding the technique, and then one day the scales drop from your eyes, something clicks inside your head and the knowledge and technique come together. Once I understood what I was doing and what being a hairdresser was all about I took to it like a demon. I ended up doing training nights like they were going out of fashion. My only fear then was missing the last train home as I got more and more engrossed in what I was doing. One night I finished at three o'clock in the morning. I think I was the only apprentice who qualified in ten months.

From the beginning I had lots of practice and experience with long hair. I became known for doing it so that it looked pretty and easy, and through experimenting with the old-fashioned setting lotions and spraying straight onto the roots I was able to get body into something that was flat before. By its very nature long hair tends to be flat on the head because its own weight pulls it down. Only if the hair is curly, or by introducing gravity-defying products, can you make it look fuller from the roots. Putting in huge rollers or using electric styling equipment helps, but unless you use gallons of hairspray it drops very quickly. Of course that was in the days before mousses, gels and volumizers were born.

Now I know that long hair is supposed to be sexy and sassy and in many cases it is. It's also supposed to be versatile – more versatile than short hair – but is it? If you think about it, the way most people use length is by getting rid of it: tying it back or putting it up.

Men are supposed to like long hair and women often keep the length for the men in their lives – but what exactly do we mean by long hair? In most cases, any head of hair that starts creeping to waist level is verging on the freaky. It does nothing but hang. Nobody needs to grow their hair any longer than about chest level. Hair that's longer than that is either little-girlie, which is unfortunate in a grown woman, or witch-like, which is downright unattractive.

I've had any number of clients come in with hair almost to the waist, asking me to do something with it 'but keep the length'. Why? Often they have terrific hair to shoulder level and after that it falls apart: it's either dry and strawlike or stringy and going into rat-tails. You've probably realized by now that I don't like it. And yet at the right length it can look terrific: as it does on such clients as Elizabeth Hurley, Jemima Khan, Jane Seymour and Kate Moss. All have long hair – it's healthy, looks terrific and has all the right versatility and attributes. Sometimes you don't even need to have hair as long as they do to get the same effect – it's all in the cutting and in the proportions. But if hair is too long it merely lies flat on the head and if it has any movement or wave its own weight will often drag the movement out.

> Far better to lop off long hair just below the shoulder, add a few layers and allow some life and movement back into it. The layers will often give a life and fullness. There's nothing you can do to really long hair without it ending up looking like a shortish cut with long bits at the end – it's a waste of both your time and money and of the stylist's time and expertise.

> Take it up to shoulder or chest level, where it will look thicker and healthier while still being long enough to be tied back into a ponytail or chignon or piled up on top of the head. A light fringe can also help balance the style. Several of my more well-known clients have had their hair trimmed to this length: Cindy Crawford and Jemima Khan, for example. And they look after their hair, too, having a trim at least every six or seven weeks.

> Certain types of hair need to be long in order to look right. Andie MacDowell, whom I first worked with when she was a model, gets away with very long hair simply because she's so beautiful. But she also has this incredibly thick, curly hair which needs a bit of length for balance. Even when she had it cut she did the right thing by keeping the layers long and chunky.

A classic Eighties look: Cindy Crawford with 'Big Hair'.

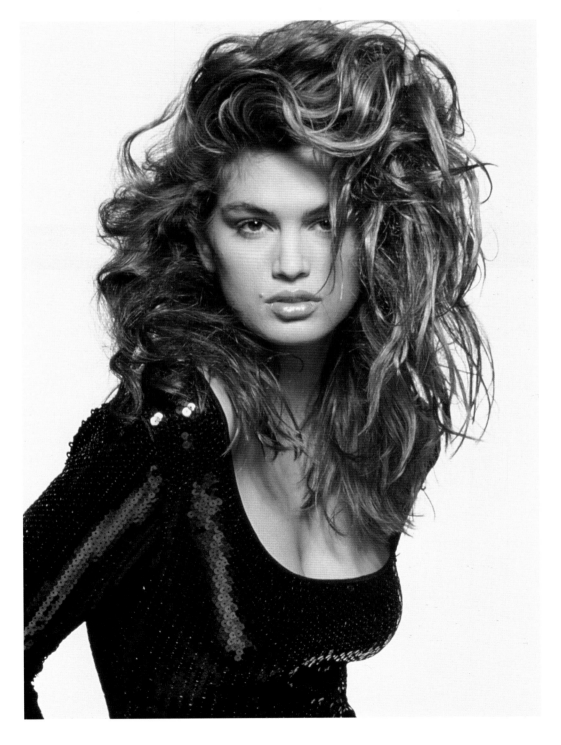

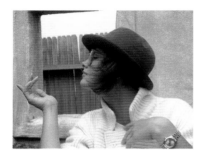

I spent quite some time in America doing shoots with Brooke Shields. At the time she was going out with Michael Jackson and needed to be heavily 'disguised' for a restaurant trip.

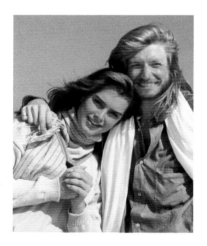

Brooke was very sweet and arranged a surprise party on the beach for my birthday, complete with chocolate cake and champagne.

Brooke Shields is another star who never lets her hair get too long. She is extremely clever at knowing when there's too much length. Throughout her years in the public eye she has managed to keep roughly the same style, yet she constantly adapts it and changes it so that it never looks dated. Of course, she's helped by having that mind-blowing big American hair that's so lustrous and wavy. I worked with her once on a fashion shoot in California – it was at the time she was going around with Michael Jackson and the poor girl was constantly pursued by press and paparazzi. She used to get quite lonely when the rest of us went off to dinner and she had to stay at the hotel to avoid being hassled. I started creating disguises for her so that she could come with us. We used a combination of hats and rolling her hair up so that it looked like a short haircut. Nobody ever guessed!

There are really no hard and fast rules these days about long and short hair provided you have the confidence in yourself, your look and your style. Those old arguments about wearing your hair short because you're older don't hold up when you consider the likes of Goldie Hawn and Diana Ross, both of whom are over fifty. If the balance and proportions as well as the shade are right for your face and skin tone, there really shouldn't be any age barrier.

It all flows from your sense of yourself and the confidence you have in your style. Having a hairdresser you can trust is a great asset in finding such a style – just as you should listen to what he says, he must also listen to you. This trust also means that neither of you is afraid to experiment at one time or another because you both have the same end in view – a better-looking you. If he says your hair is too thin or too damaged to hold a certain style, you have to believe him. If he says that a certain type of perm or colour is not right for your hair, remember that his knowledge and experience is what you're paying for.

It's been interesting to note over the past few years that both men and women are now enjoying the same freedom to choose what length to wear their hair. It demonstrates the greater confidence each gender has developed in itself. Now we can have what suits us and not what age or convention decrees. There really aren't that many rules any longer.

So, in spite of all this, suppose you want to grow your hair. It's a trying time. Hair that needed to be trimmed every five to six weeks suddenly appears to have stopped growing altogether and the whole procedure seems to take for ever. Hair grows at roughly half an inch a month (though this slows down as we get older), but most people almost immediately run out of patience when they decide to grow their hair.

Be realistic as well as patient. Don't cherish false expectations. For instance, if your hair is thick and bushy it will appear to grow outwards before it grows downwards, so that instead of having a neat style you may have a much bushier one for a while – but it helps to know this before you start. There will come a time when it begins to grow downwards and you'll start to have the effect you want. There is a way forward.

The transition phase is possibly the most depressing bit. This is when you have an outgrown version of your former style rather than a too-short version of the look you're aiming for. Hold your nerve and keep your patience. It's most often at this stage, when the new style can almost be seen, that impatience takes over and the client asks for a cut. The best approach is to try to keep the balance of your old style throughout this time. Have the bottom layers trimmed to hold the shape as the top layers grow, but don't be too drastic or the growing will take for ever. Remind yourself that all growth slows down at some stage – roughly when length reaches about 10–11 inches. It's also worth noting that hair, like plants, grows more quickly during the summer months.

If you have a fringe it often helps to keep it while you are growing the rest of your hair, just so that when you look in the mirror you can still see remnants of a familiar style that you are comfortable with. It helps you realize that the growing process is not a total disaster and once you've achieved the length you want then you can begin to let the fringe grow too or adjust it to your new style.

You may start with one style in mind, but as your hair grows and its shape changes you might change your decision. Be open-minded, and listen to what your stylist has to say. After all, this is the person who knows your hair and its needs as well as you do. This is the person who's seen you at your worst – dry hair, dull roots, fed up – but has your interests at heart and only wants you to look your best and feel great.

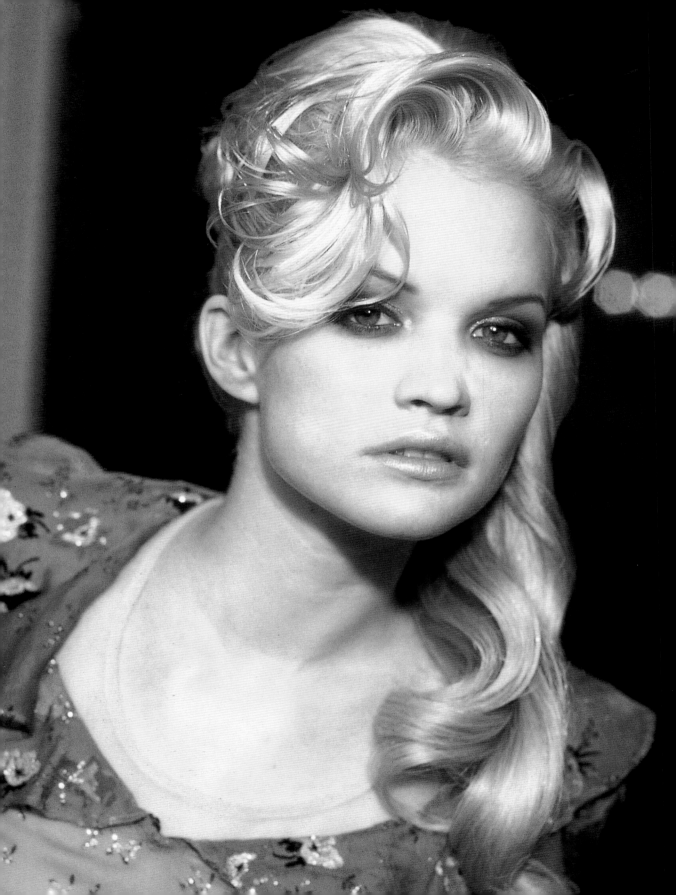

Caring for LONG HAIR

Once you have achieved the length, you need to remember that long hair behaves in a different way from short and needs different care and handling. The first thing you notice about people with long hair is that, unless like Kate Moss or Maria Shriver they are very confident, they are forever touching it. This probably started way back when they first grew it – they didn't know how to cope with it and were constantly fiddling with it, pushing it out of their eyes, off their face or behind their ears. It's a habit born out of insecurity and it pulls, stretches and tangles the hair. Long hair is much more susceptible to damage than short because its ends are further away from the nourishment coming from the roots. Be aware of how much you fiddle or mess with it and try to curtail that habit.

Secondly, be careful when your hair is wet and again try not to tamper with it too much. Hair is elastic and strong but the more you pull it the weaker it gets. When it's wet it loses up to 25 per cent of its elasticity and any further pulling, such as over-enthusiastic combing or brushing, could take it to breaking point. Use a mild shampoo, and make sure that your hair is well soaked first. If the hair is good and wet you won't need as much shampoo and you won't need to push and shove the hair while spreading the shampoo in it. Always use a conditioner, taking care to massage it well into the ends of the hair. Remove excess moisture with a towel without rubbing or dragging and only then comb it through. A wide-toothed comb is essential for this stage – never a brush, which will only pull and tangle. If you come across any tangles with the comb, hold the hair above the tangle with one hand to prevent tugging from the root and gently comb through the rest of it, working slowly and carefully. This is particularly important if you have curly hair.

A golden rule – whether you have long or short hair – is never to begin styling until the hair is 80 per cent dry. It's important to remember this with short styles, but with long ones it's paramount, because the more you play with the hair the flatter it will become. The weight of long hair is enough to keep it close to the scalp and you don't need to exacerbate that. All styles need movement, not so much to make the hair stand out but to help it look healthy and attractive. Getting movement and volume into long hair takes expertise and care, but this is made a lot easier by the many aids and products now available.

Volume begins at the root. For fine or limp hair a light root or body perm is an option. Use one of the many volumizing products on the market, such as my own Hairomatherapy Lift, Thicken and Shine spray. This has extracts of frankincense and eucalyptus alongside panthenol and polymers. For those who prefer mousse, we have a hair thickening product which gives lots of volume and hold without stickiness. Turning your head upside down to blow-dry the roots also helps, but better still is to toss your hair to each side in turn and systematically lift the roots with a vent brush or a wide-toothed comb.

Long curly hair needs different treatment from straight hair when it's wet. Whether it's coarse or fine, curly hair is often more fragile than straight. Conditioning is a must after each shampooing, and in addition a deep conditioner or masque once or twice a month. Comb in the conditioner with a wide-toothed comb, starting from the ends. After the final rinse try not to roll or twist your wet curls in a towel; simply blot out the excess moisture instead. The easiest way to begin drying and styling very curly hair is to divide it into sections and dry each one carefully. Again it's important to use a product, but this time you need to start the drying process when the hair is

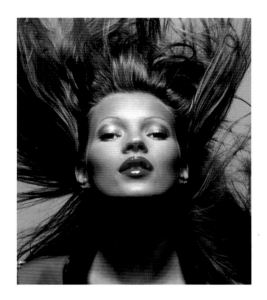

This fantastic shot of Kate Moss with long hair flying in the wind is one of my favourites.

about 50 per cent wet. The best products for curly hair are those devised to counteract frizz. My new Style and Shine Spray Serum contains natural ingredients such as bergamot and ylang ylang, which help relax the hair while the polymers are conditioning and strengthening it. This lotion also helps eliminate static. However, if you want to keep hair curly, divide it into sections but use a diffuser attachment on the dryer.

To prevent the hair that frames the face from going too flat, it's useful to put in some stand-up pin-curls or large Velcro rollers while you're drying the rest of it. People used to laugh and call me the pin-curl king when I first started to do this, but it does work and it helps soften the hair around the face. To help avoid frizz use a diffuser attachment on your hairdryer and dry from underneath the hair. Finally, when the hair is dry, take a little serum or wax and gently run through the hair, occasionally tweaking and gently pulling at individual curls or waves to give definition and a good finish.

If you have very curly as opposed to slightly wavy hair it's better for its health to dry it curly. However, this does not take into account your personal preference. Often a different cut or style, that is, longer layers, will help it appear straighter. And then strategic blow-drying, either along the hairline, the fringe, the front or the top layers, will give the illusion of smoother hair. When you want to do it yourself, use a special serum such as my Frizz Control Shine Serum or Blow-Dry Lotion, and take small sections of hair, beginning at the front, over a round brush. Dry on a medium heat. Rain and humidity are the real frizz demons but serum puts a coating on the hair that helps to repel their effects.

A little can go a long way

One of the reasons people say they like wearing their hair long is because they can do so much with it – and yet these are the same people who rarely do anything with it other than scrape it back with a scrunch. However, there are now so many different accessories that you can do quite a lot with long hair without too much effort. I believe that hair is most attractive when it doesn't look as if it's wearing its owner, so keep the more complicated styles for grand occasions and weddings. A plethora of combs, bands and clips is now available, all of which can hold hair back, help keep it up or take it to one side.

* Pins or grips are good for controlling untidy fringes or indeed for styles that are growing out.
* Slides are best for keeping whole sections of hair off your face.
* Combs are great for keeping sections of hair in place, for tidying up straggly ends if you're wearing your hair in a pleat, or merely for keeping hair off your face. They have a much softer effect than clips.
* Pin clips are best for keeping chignons and pleats in order.
* Covered elastic bands and scrunches are a gentle way of holding hair back and will not damage or tangle.
* Bands are fine for keeping hair off the face. For a more sophisticated version, use your sunglasses.

Any long style that's held back will usually look better if it's not too severe. Try to keep a tendril or curl loose, spiky bits or a knot at the back for that spontaneous feel. A touch of hairspray will help keep the rest of the style in place, but don't use too much. Be careful to use a good spray: some tend to dull the hairs instead of add shine.

And then, of course, you can always backcomb your hair. Backcombing works best on hair that's neither too silky nor too freshly shampooed because at that stage the hair is too fine to hold the tease, though a spot of hairspray helps. For this you need a fine-toothed comb – one with lots of teeth. Do the root area to about halfway down the hair shaft. Smooth over gently and spray. The great thing about backcombing is that you need only put it into the hair where you want volume.

Long Hair Lovers

These people take care of their long hair, which is why it always looks so terrific:

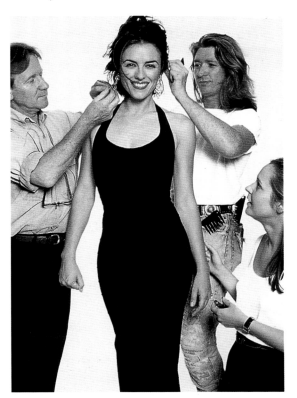

Elizabeth Hurley
Yasmin Le Bon
Maria Shriver
Jennifer Aniston
Jemima Khan
Cindy Crawford
Queen Noor of Jordan
Brooke Shields
Goldie Hawn

I was part of the team that created this Tatler *cover look with Elizabeth Hurley, which led to her winning the contract with Estée Lauder.*

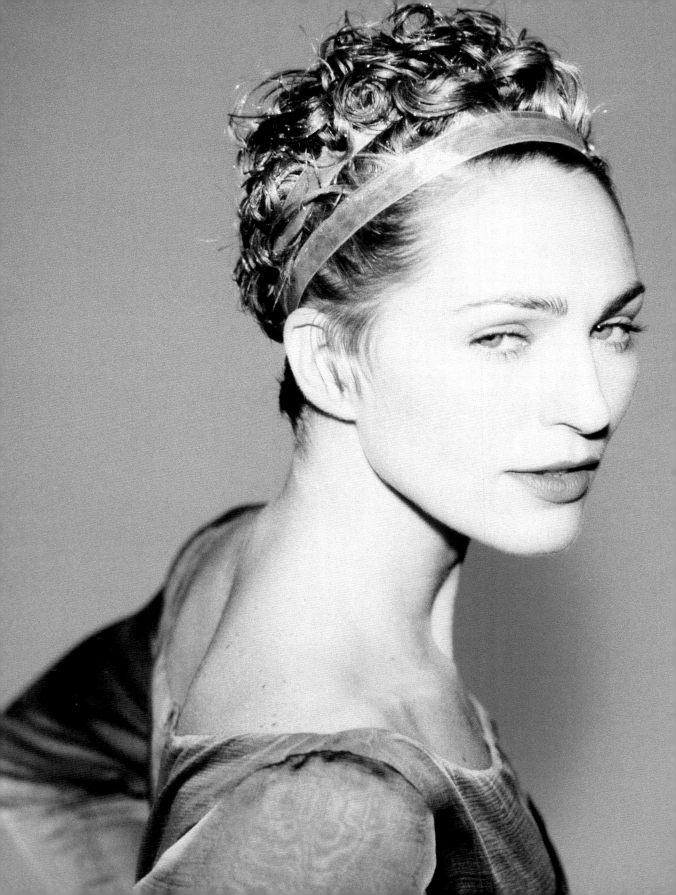

I'm better known for my shorter styles, and it's these styles that have generated the most comment.

I'd been doing the Duchess of York's hair for about eighteen months before we decided to cut it into a bob, and I'd been doing Yasmin Le Bon's hair since she was seventeen – years before I gave it the chop. Yet people only remember these short styles, along with the ones I've given to Selina Scott, Anthea Turner, Nicola Formby, Julia Carling, Amanda de Cadenet, and even to *Vogue* editor, Alexandra Shulman.

SHORT AND SWEET

When I cut Selina Scott's hair into that short, heavy-fringed style it caused more comment than any other style that year. It was on the front pages of newspapers, and pictures of it were taken into hairdressers across the country. And yet it was not appreciably shorter than before. Selina had been a client for a long time and over a period of a few months we'd been gradually taking it shorter and shorter without too much comment. I think it was a hairstyle that was right for its time. It was short, easy and yet looked sophisticated. And it made a huge change from all the big *Dallas* and *Dynasty*-type hairstyles around then.

I suppose it's hardly surprising that I'd eventually become known for my cuts – after all, it was the first type of hairdressing I ever did. When I was still at school my dad bought a hair-cutting kit through an advertisement in the *Daily Mirror*. He'd use it on us all. We'd put sheets all over the floor and furniture while he snipped away. Then I began to practise on my brothers and sisters and, as I

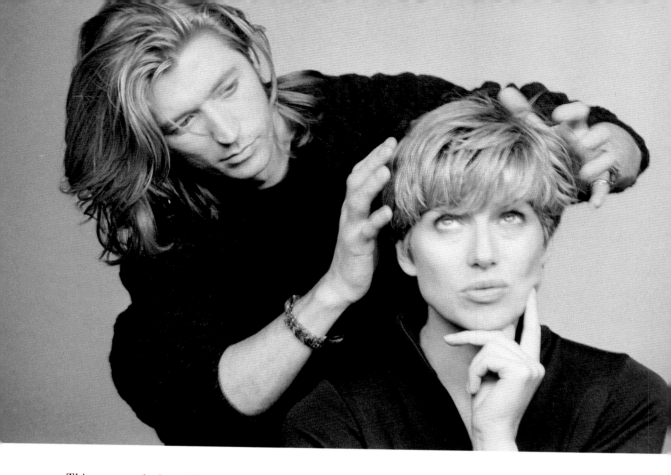

This was a style that with minimal adaptation could look good on most age groups – which is why Selina's photograph was all over the newspapers and magazines.

got bolder, on some schoolfriends too. It was all very badly done but it showed, I suppose, that I had either an interest or a facility, or both.

Oddly enough, my dad would never let me cut his hair. I would play around with it, comb in the odd quiff or whizz in the odd slick of Brylcreem, but even when I started hairdressing as a career it was quite a time before he let me touch his hair.

I'd done the style Selina had a year or so previously for a *Vogue* photographic session. People immediately liked it then – a number brought the picture into the salon and asked for the same cut. It was very short at the back and sides but heavy at the front and full on top. It was also very feminine; it had all the right ingredients. People love a short haircut that works and this one did because it suited different types and different ages. It looked great on young faces, casually sophisticated on middle-aged women and with a bit more added body could easily be worn by older women too.

It also appeared instantly accessible – you could walk into the hairdresser's and say: I want that style. It wasn't like hankering after something that was long or curly or platinum blonde – you could just go in and get it done. This one was casual but controlled, chunky but feminine on a woman who exuded a certain confidence. It wasn't girly but neither was it too sophisticated, and men loved it which meant it had masses of sex appeal. Whenever men like a short style it gets the green light and suddenly everyone wants it. This cut still has its aficionados and over the years has influenced similar styles and other stylists. I first did this for Selina in 1985/6, and eight years later the Princess of Wales was sporting a similar cut when she was photographed in a plain back polo-neck sweater by Patrick Demarchelier.

It's odd that even at the end of the twentieth century there are still stereotypical views on hair. You know the ones that say long hair is about the traditional womanly virtues, such as patience, loyalty and endurance, while short hair is about modernity and independence. But in reality there aren't any hard and fast rules about the right time to have long hair and the right time to have short.

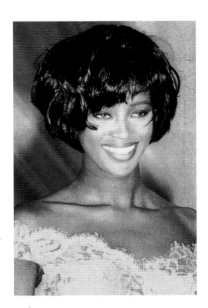

You won't see many pictures of Naomi Campbell with short hair and, yes, it is a wig!

Teenagers often opt for short hair because they had long hair throughout their childhood. Twenty-year-olds change to short styles for their jobs; the career path makes them want to appear well-groomed and in control. Most women who cut their hair in their twenties rarely grow it back because once they've got used to the ease of shorter styles it's quite difficult to get back into the swing of long hair. Women who have kept their hair long through their thirties and forties and then decide to go for short need to beware of going for something too drastic.

When I did Jilly Cooper's hair she was terrified I was going to lop the whole lot off. For years she'd been having her hair done at home by someone from the local village and she was happy with her long wavy style. Now why would I want to change that? I don't think it's the hairdresser's job to

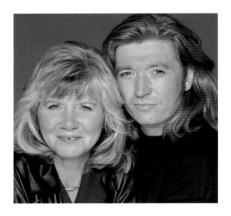

Jilly Cooper wanted to keep her length, so I made her hair look fuller with shorter layers at the top and sides while in fact shortening it to shoulder level. She was delighted.

Anthea Turner had the hairstyle everybody wanted. It was the most asked-for style in salons up and down the country – although I made it look slightly funkier for this cover shoot.

dismiss the way a client likes to look. The problem with Jilly's hair was that it was just a bit too long, a little too straggly, and it needed tidying up. It also needed to be given some shape, which it had lost over the years. By the time I'd finished with it, although it was shorter it still looked long, and it had shape and movement. I'd also softened the fringe and the rather heavy layers she had around the crown. It would have looked even better if those layers had been longer, but a hairdresser can't add length – only the illusion of it. Everybody loved it and that's all you could want as a hairdresser.

Although Selina's style was the one to hit the headlines, the most successful throughout the country was Anthea Turner's. While Selina's was flattering, it did demand more from the wearer, possibly because it was that much shorter. All types and ages felt immediately at home with Anthea's style – I've even done it on a sixty-year-old. Every so often one of the trade papers does a survey on what people want at their hairdressers. The styles that people are after are those worn by Anthea Turner, Jennifer Aniston, Liz Hurley, Julia Carling, Meg Ryan and Helena Christensen. All of these apart from Meg Ryan and Jennifer Aniston are my clients, and Anthea's is still the number one.

I did the prototype of that style on a society girl but it was not noticed so much because she didn't have Anthea's profile or Anthea's timing. Like most things, if the timing is right for a style or a change then you're halfway there. Anthea had a lot of exposure on TV, she's pretty, bubbly and unthreatening, but most of all she's very showbiz, very eyes and teeth, and people love her for it. She's accessible and acceptable to everyone, and she's also the right

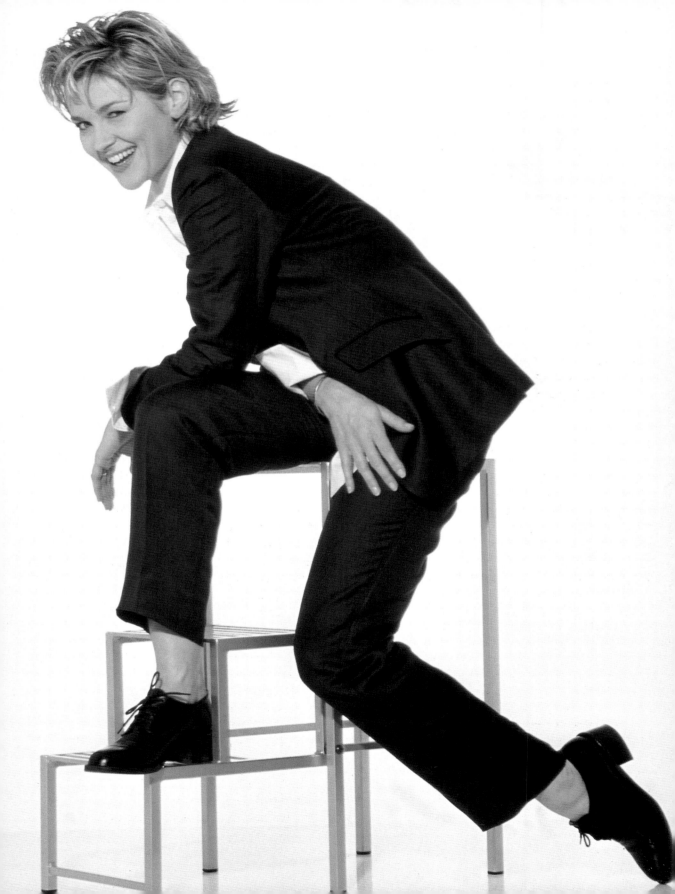

age: neither too young nor too old. Her style was a style whose time had come. And it's one that suits most people, apart from those with exceptionally frizzy, curly hair.

It was also a style that broke a television rule. Anthea was the first anchorwoman not to have anchorwoman hair. Most TV styles have to go through the rigorous assessment of the lighting cameraman and what he does not want and will not have is see-through. If you look carefully at most TV performers' hairstyles you will not be able to see anything through them. They are neat and very clean in line. That's why the layered bob is one of the most popular of all the telly styles.

Anthea's cut is quite the opposite – it's all see-through. She completely broke the mould. It's a fairly standard layered look, although the layers are cut in quite a choppy way, more chunky than subtle, and then I feathered it. This is simply a case of taking the last three-quarters of an inch of each section and thinning it. But it's not the usual sort of thinning, where the hair can be left looking and feeling too stringy. This is a light and gentle feathering. It softens the edges and gives the haircut that lightness all the way around. After that I add some product to the top to give it body – some mousse or a styling spray – and then blow-dry it, putting a little kick into the ends.

People have a misconception about short hair – that you can only wear it one way. But you can in fact change it quite a lot. That's true of Anthea's style, for instance, and it's the same with most short looks. You can make a short style curlier with rollers, pin-curls or tongs, straighter by blow-drying it that way, change the effect by moving the parting, style it away from the face, or indeed bring more hair on to the forehead in a thicker fringe. When I did a cover shoot with Anthea for *Tatler* we kept it fairly standard, but then we made it much funkier for the pictures inside. Using gel or wax it's easy to give any style a harder, spikier edge. Anthea looks sophisticated with it worn like this rather than her more usual girl-next-door persona.

There's probably nobody less like the girl next door than Yasmin Le Bon, whose hair I've been doing for years and years. She has incredible hair: thick, heavy, silky with the most fantastic shine, which is why she is ideal for those hair product ads. On the other hand it's quite difficult to handle because it has a very soft texture – not that anybody would complain if they had her sort of hair. When she said she wanted a complete change I think it was because she'd got bored, like everyone does after a long time of having the same look, and she probably decided she was grown-up enough to give the long straight version a rest for a while.

It wasn't the first time we'd cut her hair, but it was the most dramatic. First of all I made it blonde, partly to effect a complete change of look and partly to rough up the

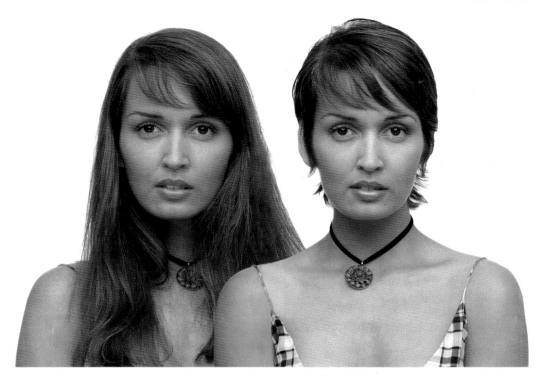

Supermodel Gail Elliot really went for the chop!

texture a bit. Then I cut it, keeping the top layers quite long while underneath the hair was layered and feathered. This allowed her to wear the style in a very grungy fashion – after all, this was in 1992 – or smooth it over for a sleek bob, or go wild and do a quiff like an old rocker, which looked fantastic. Again it was a much-copied style. People went into their hairdresser's and asked for the look – probably more than anything because they liked Yasmin and the way she looked and had never seen her with a short cut before.

It was probably when I did the Duchess of Kent for *Vogue* that people began to comment on my ability to soften and enhance quite severe and stylized looks. Up until then many people had thought my styles were only brought about in a studio or salon on models, actresses and television stars. With the Duchess they saw that I could make the styles work on real people too, and people of all ages. For years the Duchess had had the same hairstyle – a classic bob with just enough length and weight to put up when she needed to for tiaras, hats or diadems. It always looked neat and elegant, but I felt it had too much of the helmet about it – too hard and stiff. I wanted to loosen it up a little, make it softer, put a little kick into the finish. She has beautiful hair, quite strong with a slight wave, and what's more she's a true natural blonde. When I suggested that we take it shorter and make it slightly softer she was a little resistant to begin with. After all, she has very definite ideas about how she likes to look and has over the years created her own style. In the end, however, she agreed, and the look was stunning: here was a middle-aged woman, a senior member of the royal family, looking like no royal had ever looked before in an Armani trouser suit and a short blonde crop. The *Vogue* spread was picked up everywhere and reproduced in all the newspapers.

A slightly funkier and even shorter version of that style was one I devised for Julia Carling – another one that's proved popular in the copying stakes. It's a sporty, easy look, whose foundation is a good basic cut. It's the sort of style that you can finger dry but which will also glam up if you add mousse, a few pin-curls and a couple of Velcro rollers. Or you can make it sharper and funkier by taking a little wax through the ends to give it an edge.

Julia is a great client and we get on extremely well. She is very lively and funny and although I've only been doing her hair for a few years she very quickly got to the stage where she trusted me and my judgement, which is why she came to me for the look I'm known for. Her hair is that English mousy type that takes colour so well, so the first thing we did was lighten it with a tint and bleach. Recently we've begun to put in very fat and obvious highlights along the front, the sort the Americans call skunk stripes, which gives it an even more glamorous appeal. One of the reasons it's become such a popular style throughout the country is that it epitomizes the easy, sporty, sexy look that's very Nineties. Nobody wants to be seen being worn by a hairstyle. Most people want to look great without too much effort, confident without too much fuss. And for all of that you have to begin with the cut.

It's extraordinary how the sports look has infiltrated our lives. Whoever thought, even a few years ago, that trainers and anoraks would be hurtling down the catwalks of Paris and Milan – even though the anoraks are made of cashmere and silk – and that every designer from Chanel to Prada would have their own version of that look. And of course you have to have the hair that goes with it. Ever since Jane Fonda came on the scene with her aerobics, women have wanted a sportier style, and their choice of haircuts has reflected that. The healthy, athletic shape is very attractive, but a woman still wants to retain her femininity too – and that comes across in her hair. Occasionally people go too far with their training and end up with too muscular a body, which doesn't look good with feminine clothes or even feminine hairstyles. At the 1998 Oscars, for instance, Madonna wore her hair long and wavy but showed off too many muscles in her sleeveless gown – it was a look that jarred.

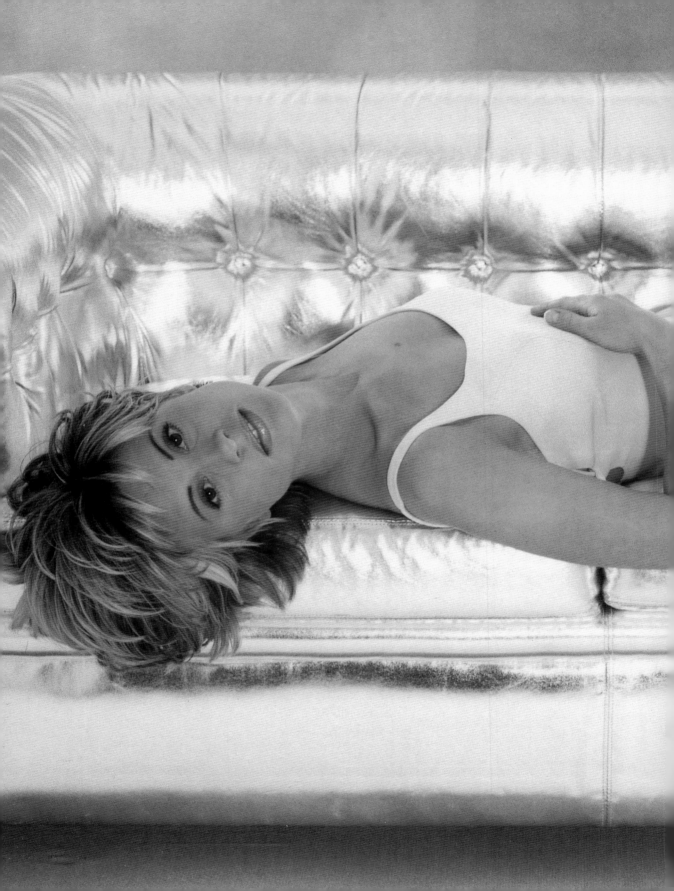

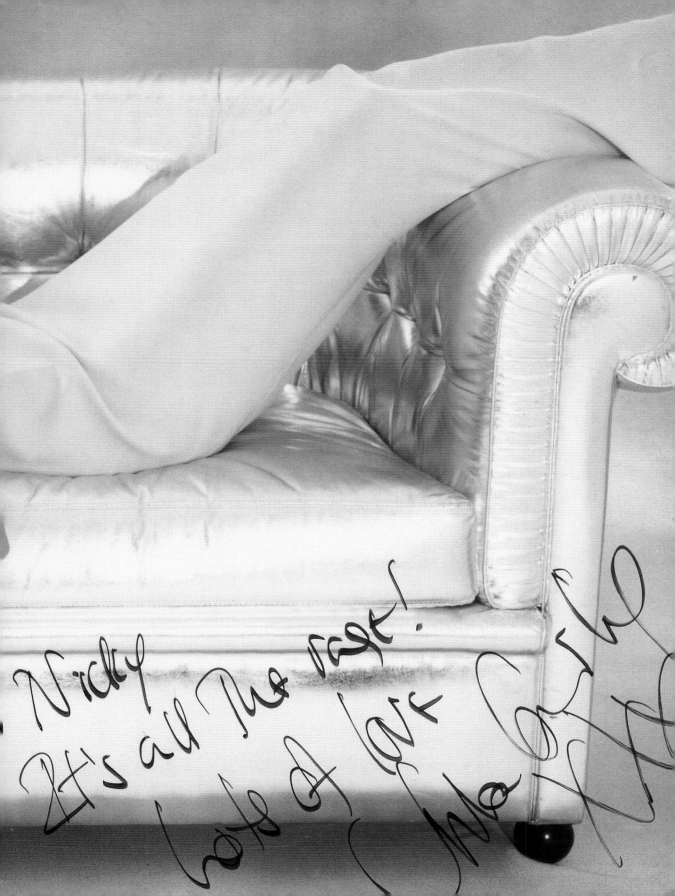

The whole sports-fashion movement has brought with it an easier, no-nonsense approach to beauty. But the more casual – albeit elegantly casual – a woman may want to appear, the more she demands from her hair. She wants it to look good, look healthy, look sexy, be no trouble – she wants a miracle every day. She's on a constant search for the ideal low-maintenance style. Perhaps Julia's style is so popular because it epitomizes this.

I'm a great advocate of short hair, but I can sometimes get it wrong. Such an occasion was when Kate Beckinsale was sent in for a cut by the director of an art-house film she was going to be working on in Spain. I knew Kate's hair and loved her look – but this was one of the days from hell. It took us seven hours to finish and by that stage I was not a happy hairdresser. Her hair was almost shoulder length and it's good, strong, slightly Asian hair with a bit of bend in it – that was to be the sticking point. Kate is beautiful, with a great face, so almost any style suits her. However, as I started to cut it, I knew I wanted to have it quite short but in a bitty, slightly messy style. She loved it but then decided she wanted it shorter. I resisted at first, but she became more insistent and I gave in. A nightmare had begun. As I made it shorter I realized that the texture of her hair was such that the minute it got really short it went dead straight and stuck out at right angles.

I knew this was not going to be right for the film, so we permed bits of it to put in some contours and shape. All the time I was doing it I thought my reputation was going to be shot to pieces. I knew that when she was filming in Spain they would have to work on her hair constantly for continuity. Even after seven hours I was unhappy about it, but there was nothing else I could do and I knew I would never see her again.

It was one of those occasions when I should have stuck to what I felt was right and what I knew her hair was capable of. I should have been the dictatorial hairdresser. I didn't see her again for months – eight, to be precise. Then she reappeared at the salon and made me do the same thing all over again, without the perm. She wanted her hair as short as possible because she loved what I'd done. But when I finished I still didn't think it was right, even though she kept the style for *Shooting Fish*. Even *Vogue* loved it, referring to it as 'a cute new Nicky Clarke crop'. Eventually, a few months later, she agreed with me, admitting she had no idea why she'd insisted on having the cut for the second time when all she did was spend hours plastering products all over it. Anyway, she still has short hair but it's now long enough to allow some movement into it and it looks wonderful.

And then there was the woman whose hair I wouldn't cut! The newspaper headline ran WHY NICKY CLARKE WOULDN'T CUT MY HAIR. It was Marie Helvin. She and her best mate Jerry Hall had gone on about whether they should have their hair cut every time I saw them, but because they were undecided we did nothing about it – until the next time we met when the discussion would start all over again.

I've known Marie for years and done her hair since the Seventies, when she wore it really straight. She went curly in the Eighties when the fashion was for big hair and this slightly gypsyish style suited her. Not so long ago she asked me to cut it again, and I agreed to so long as she let me straighten it so that it looked slightly smoother and more spontaneous – otherwise it would have looked like a slightly shorter version of her long style. She likes her curls, though, so we decided not to go ahead.

But Marie did subsequently go ahead – to another hairdresser who made her look fantastic with a great short style reminiscent of Ava Gardner. When one of the newspapers saw it they did some great pictures and a story about why I wouldn't cut it short!

why nicky clarke wouldn't cut my hair

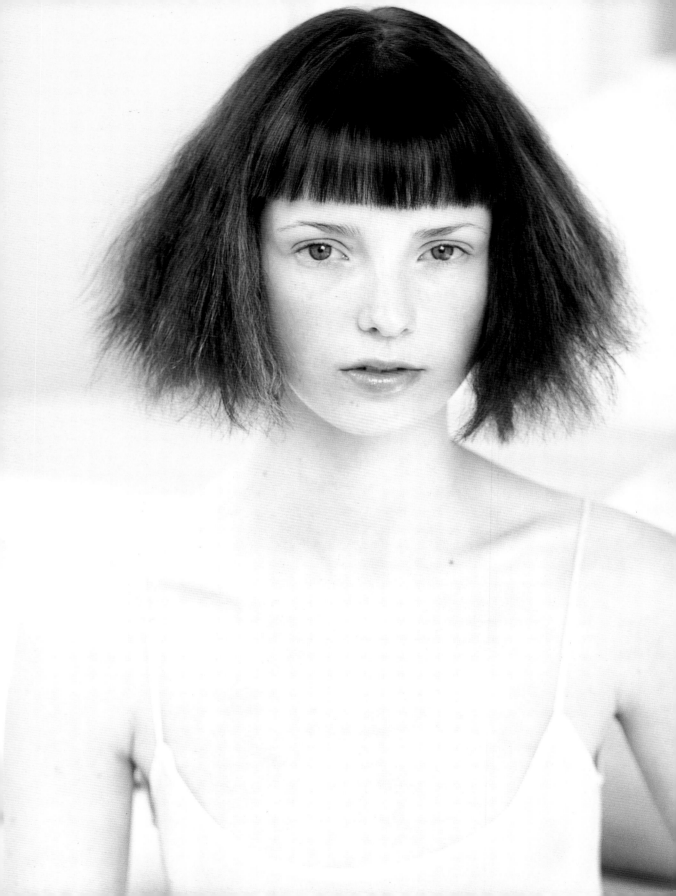

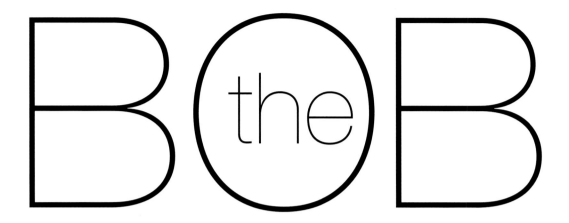

One of the greatest short
styles ever has been the bob,
which has been around in one
form or another since the
Ancient Egyptians. True
enough, Cleopatra wore hers
quite long, but mostly the
classic bob is anywhere from
shoulder level upwards. It's one
basic shape but with hundreds
of variations. We can trace it
from paintings of Tudor
monarchs to Josephine Baker
in the early part of this
century, with her slicked-back
short and wavy version, and
all the way to today.

However, the bob came into its own in this century in the Twenties with Louise Brooks's dark, shiny, fringed version. Compared with the complicated Edwardian styles that had gone before it, this was seriously low-maintenance – very easy to do and to look after. It was one of those great styles that just works with gravity: the hair falls naturally and doesn't have to perform any gravity-defying tricks or curls. It coincided with a complete change in fashion, too – to a simpler look along straight geometric lines as whalebones, bodices and a myriad petticoats were thrown out.

The popularity of the bob also coincided with the rise of the Marcel wave and so part of its charm was that it could be worn straight or wavy. It reached its style zenith in the Thirties with Coco Chanel, who never wore her hair any other way and was to influence how women were to look and dress for the rest of the century. During the Forties it became rather stiff and set as styles grew more elaborate. Barbara Stanwyck had a wonderful version, as did Joan Crawford. During the Fifties it was set with a big wave but it held a strong appeal as women went to the hairdressers clutching photographs of Doris Day.

During the Sixties and early Seventies the bob was completely re-invented by Vidal Sassoon, with his five-point cut. While this was modern and avant-garde, those early Vidal styles still required a good bit of backcombing. Early pictures of Cilla Black's bob show how backcombed and lacquered it needed to be. I suppose the most stylish exponents of it at that stage were Biba and Mary Quant, and almost forty years later Quant still hasn't felt the need to change her hairstyle, although she has adapted it over time: it's now softer with more movement.

During the Seventies it got confused with the pageboy and a sort of hybrid appeared, ranging from the quite long, layered bob to the really short Purdey style that was created for Joanna Lumley in *The Avengers*. Now while I cannot claim to have created that style, I was there when it happened at Leonard. The prototype was cut in about 1974 on a blonde model and was much looser than the one that eventually turned up on television. Joanna was sent to Leonard by the studios in 1976. He adapted the cut for her hair, which is very thick and strong and quite wavy. He blow-dried it quite strongly to straighten it but he also brushed it slightly to the side. However, once it got into the hands of the studio hairdresser, it was turned into more of a pudding-bowl cut – Leonard's's version was much more flattering.

At about the same time we saw the rise of the stacked perm bob – with the perm underneath the top layers to give the hair volume and make it stand out. Sonia Rykiel was the person best known for her stacked version, and she still wears roughly the same style. What is fantastic about the bob is that it constantly reinvents itself –

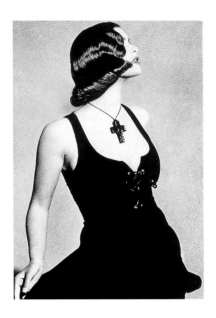

Linda Evangelista alone has reinvented it three or four times using different lengths, colours and fringes. The editor of American *Vogue*, Anna Wintour, has turned it into a modern-day classic and is never seen with a hair out of place, while model Karen Elson has sported the post-modern version: with her bright-red tint and very short fringe it looks new and yet very *Parisienne*. Fashion legend Diana Vreeland's bob was timeless with its patent-leather scraped-back look, while Suzy Menkes from the *Herald Tribune* adds gravity-defying quiffs to her classic cut to give it her own personal twist.

Mostly, however, the bob is perennially popular because it works and it's easy. And like many short styles, looking after it has become easier and easier with the advent of so many styling products. Ever since new products first started to appear in the late Seventies they've changed the way we do our hair and the demands we make on it. The old, complicated type of hair maintenance with perms and sets was no longer necessary. Mousse brought a freshness and spontaneity to the way we styled.

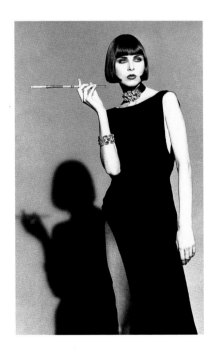

I'd been working and experimenting with products throughout my working life, particularly on session work in the studio. When you're working to create photographs you're constantly on the lookout for something that will give a different texture, a slicker finish, a faster result. Any time I went out of the country I combed chemists and drugstores and brought back whatever I could find. I'd start mixing them together to see what effect they'd have. In the very early days I used to work with an old setting lotion that came in small phials. For normal usage you emptied one onto the hair, combed it through

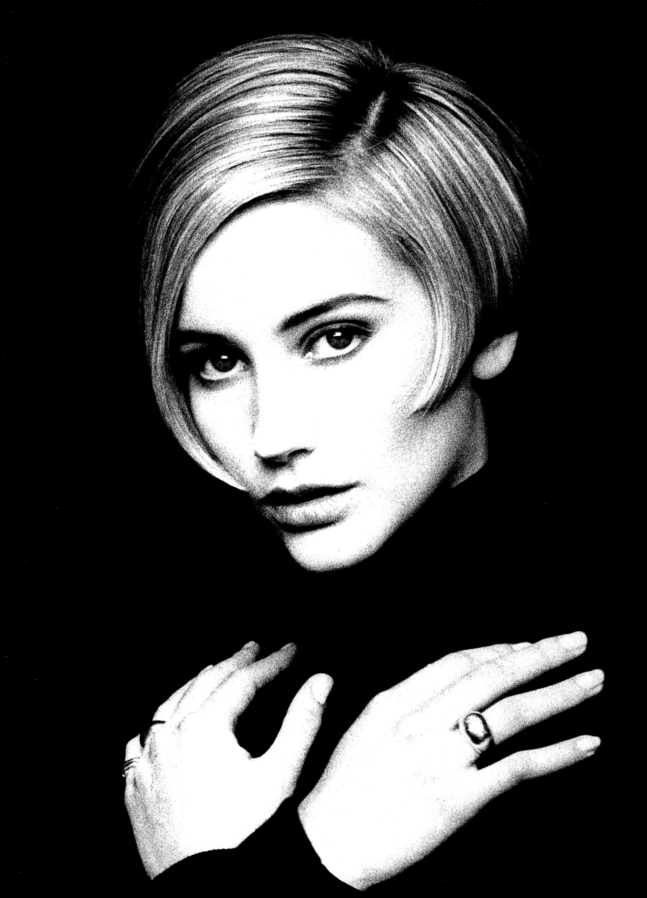

and set it. But I used to get a whole load of them, empty them into a spray bottle, and concentrate the spray where I wanted volume, lift and body. Often it was a matter of spritzing a lot onto the roots, a bit on the mid-length and hardly any on the ends. This way I immediately got the desired effect. I was able to defy gravity with all that root lift. At the time it was quite revolutionary and I was pleased with myself!

Before mousse appeared most hairstyles were basically flat. Even the Farrah Fawcett style was flat at the roots and raised only with the flicks at the end. Mousse changed all that when it first appeared in 1980. At about the same time I began bringing wax back from trips to the States. Wax had been developed for the Afro market, where it was used to straighten hair. I used it mostly to give texture to different styles. When I was working on editorial shoots for major fashion magazines, I'd often use mousse, allow the hair to dry naturally and then almost sculpt the shape with wax.

FIVE GOOD REASONS TO GO SHORT

1. If you have fine hair and it's long it will eventually start to look limp and lifeless. But if you go short with layers it immediately looks more luxurious, thicker and more shapely.
2. A good short cut will highlight your features. No-one can see what great cheekbones, fine eyes or elegant neck you have if they're constantly hidden behind curtains of hair.
3. You'll have more time. Shorter hair is easier to manage and quicker to dry.
4. There'll be fewer bad hair days because there are fewer things to go wrong with a short style. Sure, if you have long hair and a bad day you can scrape it off your face – but that's not a style.
5. A totally different shorter cut will give you a whole new image. You'll look at both your wardrobe and your make-up in a much fresher way.

WHEN TO GO SHORT

- When you fancy a change.
- Ignore all those strictures about age: short can be sexy on the young, elegant on the middle-aged and carefree on the elderly.
- When you want to take control, either of your life, your job, or both, and you don't want to mess about with complicated styles. Short hair is sharp and means business.
- When you understand that there's more than one way to wear a short hairstyle – a good stylist will show you the permutations. If he or she doesn't, then *ask*.
- When you know you have the confidence and ability to be able to look after it without worrying or wasting time.
- When you're feeling good about yourself – short hair makes more of a statement about you than even a change of colour.

HOW TO GET THAT GREAT SHORT CUT

- Talk, talk and talk to your stylist, who should be able to recommend possible and probable styles.
- Tell him or her why you want to go short. It's important for your stylist to be able to understand your reasons.
- Tell your stylist how much time you want to spend looking after it.
- Look at photographs of short styles you like and discuss which would work best on you.
- Don't discount a colour change at the same time. As was the case of Yasmin Le Bon, your hair texture might need a little 'roughing' up to hold a shorter style. Chemical changes in the hair often give it more body. Don't worry: it's the texture not the condition that needs this roughing treatment.
- Don't rush into making a decision. If you're still unsure, stick with your usual style for the time being. Most decisions made in haste are regretted, but at least you'll have started the dialogue between you and your hairdresser.
- Once it's done – don't panic. All change takes a little time to get used to.
- Remember, if you really hate it, it's not the end of the world. You can start growing it straight away!

WHAT MAKES A GREAT CUT

- One that works. It sounds obvious, but it's surprising how many short cuts don't work and take far too much time and effort to look after.
- One that works with the way your hair is. You may hanker after a smooth, sleek style but if your hair is coarse and curly you're going to spend hours – sometimes futile ones – trying to keep to a smooth style.
- One that has the minimum work attached to it.
- One that's versatile. With a change of product or a different technique you can change it around.
- One that makes you feel comfortable because it suits you and gives you the look you want.

THE JOY
OF
COLOUR

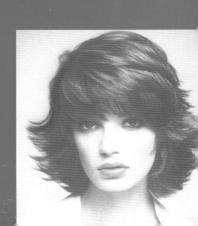

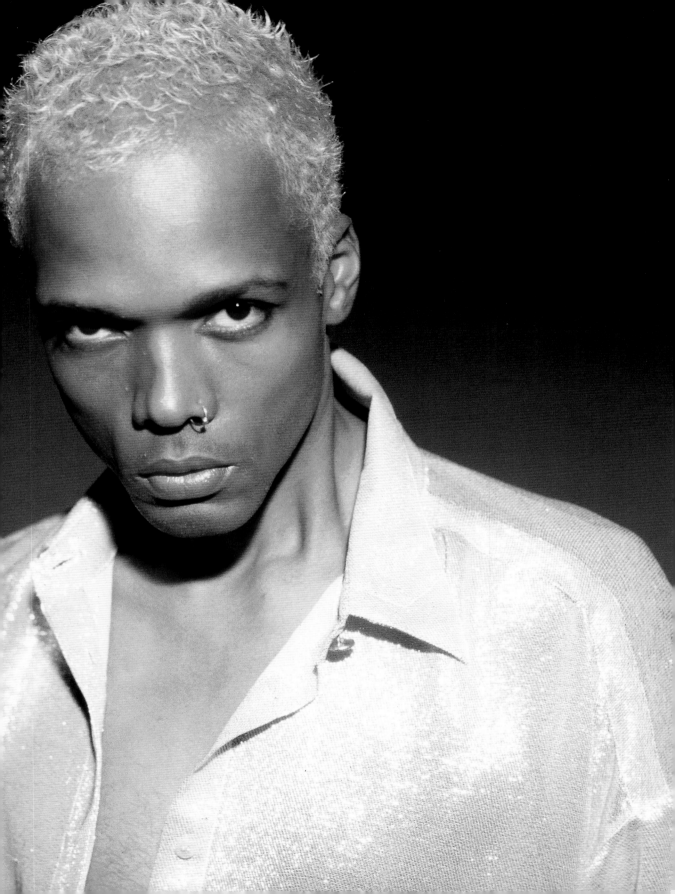

More people than ever are changing their hair colour and what is especially surprising is the number of men doing it. The colours available now are more natural than they've ever been before, and that's probably what makes them attractive to men. It was people like Bryan Ferry who paved the way for guys to use colour in their hair. Punk showed up the potential of exotic colour change, while rockers like Rod Stewart were the first to go for highlights in an attempt to show that blonds really do have more fun. We see it now with David Beckham and Brad Pitt. But in general, men are probably at the stage women were at ten to fifteen years ago.

Today women are much more knowledgeable about what products can do and what they want from them. They recognize that colorants are so technologically advanced that if they don't like the colour they've chosen they can change it to something else almost immediately. They also have the nous to know that too many extreme colour changes can have an adverse effect on their hair. But mostly people stay within the range of shades that suits them – be it blonde, red or brunette.

Another great attitude breakthrough is that women now have the confidence to have their colour as natural or as unnatural as they want. There's absolutely no stigma about it, though there was some about twenty years ago. On the other hand, there's nothing new about wanting to change the colour of our hair. Most women begin by thinking Mother Nature knows best, but in the precocious that lasts until they're about nine and in the rest of the female population until they've hit their teens.

Before chemicals were invented natural methods were the only ones available; henna has to be the oldest hair cosmetic of all. How many young girls wasted time and energy trying to lighten bits of their hair in the sun with lemon juice and occasionally vodka! The breakthrough came earlier in this century when the powerful force of bleaching was first encountered. The birth of the platinum blonde was one of the main hair turning points of the century – before bleach you really had to be born blonde. But once its efficacy was established there was no holding back the numbers of women who wanted to be blonde. Their heroines were Mae West, Jean Harlow, Jayne Mansfield and the blonde icon herself, Marilyn Monroe. The constant retouching, the root work and the overbleaching must have done terrible things to hair health and condition, but the end result was too much in demand for anybody to care. Somebody once told me that Diana Dors had her roots retouched every few days. Along the way rinses were developed to soften the often harsh shades of orange and yellow that too much bleach brought about, and gradually a softer type of blonde appeared on the scene: the Kim Novak and Doris Day shades of blonde, the creamy beige and the soft gold. Alongside this, however, came one of the more bizarre washes of the lot: the blue rinse. Fine for a short while if it's subtle, but heaved on with little thought for the after-effect it was almost ghoulish. It certainly dimmed the brassiness but it had all the attractiveness of neon.

At first such drastic colour changes were frowned upon in certain sections of society. Snobbery said that it was all right for actresses and dancers but not for women who were going to be wives and mothers. But the women who were going to be wives and mothers had their own views. As soon as the propaganda machine got going, saying that blondes had more fun, there was no stopping the flood. It's also worth

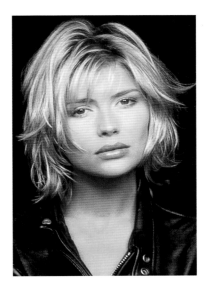

Great advances have been made in hair colour since the days when it was bleach and peroxide and hair felt like straw. Now there are many ways of achieving a look while maintaining the hair's condition.

remembering that blonde, or rather the right shade of blonde, is an immensely flattering colour, particularly to pale and creamy skins. Changing the colour of your hair is a bold and confident statement, even if it's a subtle change. A woman who makes a drastic change in the colour of her hair is making more than a statement. This is someone who wants or needs to get rid of what was there before, or is making an attempt to be someone different. For instance, take a pretty French brunette in the mid-Fifties who'd made a couple of films that had been quietly noted. One day she decided to go blonde and before the world knew what was happening a phenomenon called Brigitte Bardot had arrived. The effect she had not just in Europe but worldwide was electrifying, and her influence can be felt and seen in every generation of babes from then on. BB was the archetypal babe.

Take another example. See what happened in the Seventies when a mousy-haired singer with a gravelly voice was just one of the band until he took to the bleach. Then 'Do Ya Think I'm Sexy' Rod Stewart began to turn out the hits and thousands of clones. Wherever he appeared he had a blonde on his arm. He could almost have been crowned King Blond. Even more important, in the world of hairdressing, he not only turned out million-selling records but he gave men permission to walk into a salon and ask for a colour change. Before Rod, 'real men' didn't dye their hair. Before Rod, they thought tin foil was for turkeys. Before Rod, they'd rather have sawn off their right foot than be seen sitting in a salon with aluminium envelopes in their hair. But once this archetypal good-time lad who loved beer and football decreed it was OK to have streaks, men began queueing up to have their hair done. (They even took to wearing Lycra.)

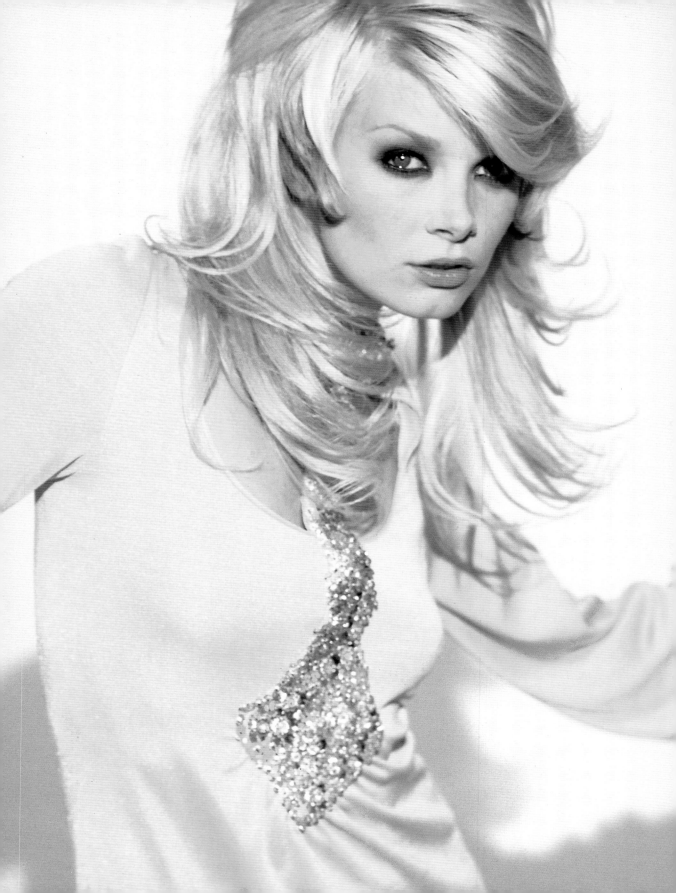

The Seventies was the

decade that began to transform what we looked for in colour and also how we achieved it. Just as the Eighties saw the growth and sophistication of styling products, in the Seventies it was the proliferation of new, sophisticated methods of colouring and bleaching that led to most of the major changes in hairdressing. It was the start of the 'natural' lights, and the beginning of the all-American blonde look that was epitomized on the covers of *Cosmopolitan*. Big, healthy, sexy girls with big, healthy, sexy and invariably blonde hair. The type of hair that Christie Brinkley had: long, windswept and glossy. The crowning glory of Lauren Hutton: a cooler shade of New York sophistication. But more than anything it was the California-sunkissed look sported by Farrah Fawcett that spread throughout the world. Millions wanted not only the flicked-back Farrah style but the colour too, complete with shine and sunkissed streaks on top of the blonde. Highlights were hair heaven.

Sure, there had been 'streaks', as they were called, before then, but they had either been crudely done or merely restricted to one or two dramatic-looking stripes in the front of the hair as worn at various times by both Anne Bancroft and Audrey Hepburn. Both were brunettes and both had almost white skunk stripes – just one or two – at the front of their hair.

Once the demand was there and once hairdressers got more proficient at highlighting, new products and new methods were developed. The first innovation was the cap, a tight-fitting latex or thin rubber bathing-cap lookalike with hundreds of little holes punched in it. Through these holes fine strands of hair were pulled by something resembling a crochet hook. It was reasonably effective (and is still used) but a little haphazard because the colourist could not really gauge where the hair was coming from – which part of the head and in what quantity. It was a bit of a hit-and-miss colouring process.

A few years later a much more sophisticated method was developed: the tin-foil packet or envelope. This has the advantage of getting very close to the root while at the same time allowing two or three or even more different shades of lights to be put in. The more sophisticated the technique, the practitioner, the product and the consumer, the more evident it became that hair is not made up of one shade alone. In its natural state one head of hair can have six, seven or more different shades and this is what gives it its depth. In the early days of colouring we only knew how to put on a flat shade, which is why blondes in particular had such a problem with the health and condition of their hair. More and more bleach was used and it was difficult, when working on regrowth, to stop bleach going onto the already bleached hair. On some heads hair had bleach dolloped on it about a dozen times. No wonder it snapped off and looked and felt like straw.

Even today it's still surprising that people don't realize that to show contrast you must have a few shades. Highlighting is a costly process not just because of the skill of a really good colourist but also because it's time-consuming. However, highlights need to be done only about every two to three months.

The great thing about lights, be they high or low, is that the permutations are endless. Once you recognize that, there are only three things to consider: the colour you put on, the thickness of the lights, and their frequency. Then you can build in as many or as few shades as you want to create your own look. You can have powerful colour done finely, or the reverse. You can even choose thick stripes in a number of shades. Whatever your choice, lights enhance the hair, adding depth, colour and texture.

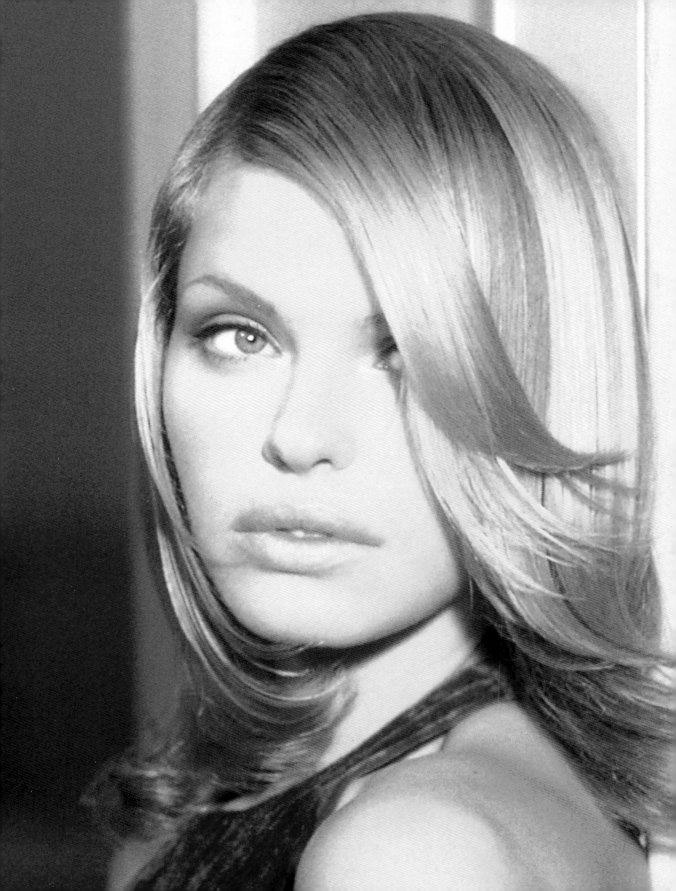

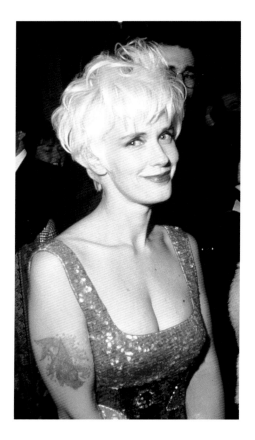

Paula Yates has always nurtured that high-maintenance look. Very short, very blonde and punky – it's a look that became her trademark.

Even overall colour tints have evolved to a new level of sophistication. They have a translucency that was not available even a few years ago. Today, there's no such thing as a flat look: the translucent effect not only allows natural shades to come through but adds depth and life to the hair. Further interest can be created with a few bleached highlights in a few key places around the front and crown to make it look as if the sun has caught the hair.

If the natural look is not for you, then you don't have to have it. If you want pink hair, like Zandra Rhodes, you're going to get it; if you want a few purple stripes, that's no problem. Blue-black could be one woman's choice, while if it's white-blonde you want, follow the Madonna and Paula Yates route.

Paula is a prime example of someone with definite ideas about her look. When I first met her, she was seventeen and had already adopted the look that she has maintained in various guises ever since. This was in the late Seventies. Her hair was bleached white and at this stage was dry and strawlike because harsh bleach had been used on her fine hair. I knew instantly that this was one person who wouldn't listen to advice about her dry ends but would look the way she wanted to. We hit it off instantly because I didn't patronize her; I understood what she was about and if she wanted this white-blonde, funky look then I was going to give her that look – while attempting to improve the condition of her hair as we went along. Sometimes it worked, sometimes it didn't. The one time she went grungy brown (not by me: I was on holiday at the time!) she didn't like it – she said nobody had noticed her.

One day a memorable phone call came from Paula from Los Angeles. She was frantic: she had overdone the bleaching, and the sunshine, and her hair had started to break off. (Something you must realize, if you're going for that strong bleached look, is that you're taking your hair to an extreme.) I told her not to worry, to keep her hair out of the sun and to get to me as quickly as she could on her return. A few days later we chopped most of it off to make it short and punky. That look became her trademark for a good few years. It's a terrific look – but seriously high-maintenance.

Now, of course, it's quite different. It's still blonde but much softer. No peroxide: it's done with a high-lift tint which gives it a nice buttery softness – a softness echoed in the style, which, although still short at the back, is longer on top.

The great advances in hair colour have been both demanded and spearheaded by women who were young in the Sixties: the babyboomers, the generation that changed the world. They were the generation that almost invented youth, the first to have the choice of careers and babies. In their thirties they were starting up their own companies alongside bringing up families.

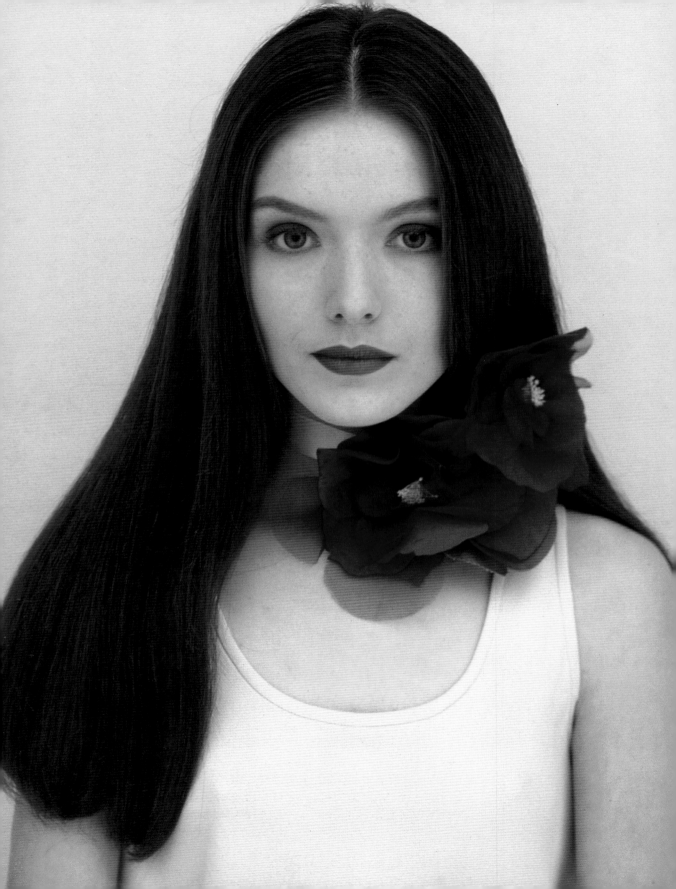

They had economic power, freedom and, most of all, the energy and will to change. When they turned forty they had Jane Fonda to show them how to firm and maintain their bodies and Giorgio Armani and Azzedine Alaia to clothe them. They were healthier and fitter than any generation before them. No way they were going to give in to one of the great signposts of age: grey hair. They remember how their mothers looked at the age of forty and fifty and firmly decided that the look didn't have a lot going for it. They were and are the great experimenters and they have taken an entire industry along with them.

Some women – a stylish few – make a statement with their grey hair. These are often women who lost their colour pigment when quite young, saw that it could carry a certain panache and decided to make a virtue out of necessity. Polly Mellen on American *Vogue*, Evangeline Blahnik, sister of super cobbler Manolo, and Christian Lacroix's favourite model and muse Marie Seznec – they all are modish and have immense presence. But it takes buckets of confidence to carry off.

Most of us start to lose the colour pigment from our hair in our early thirties. By the time we hit our fifties, on average around half the hairs on our head are grey. Many women hardly even know they have grey hairs because their usual colorants keep the offending hairs hidden. But even those to whom it comes as a shock have no need to worry. There are several different ways of coping with the grey. You can disguise it with temporary rinses or vegetable colours, both of which wash out after about six shampoos. A semi-permanent colour will last longer – up to about twenty shampoos – but you need to watch re-growth around the parting. Highlights and lowlights are extremely effective. They blur the colour contrasts between the grey and the other shades. Even better, they need re-doing only every two to three months.

For those who like the idea of grey hair, a number of special products are available that take the dinginess out of

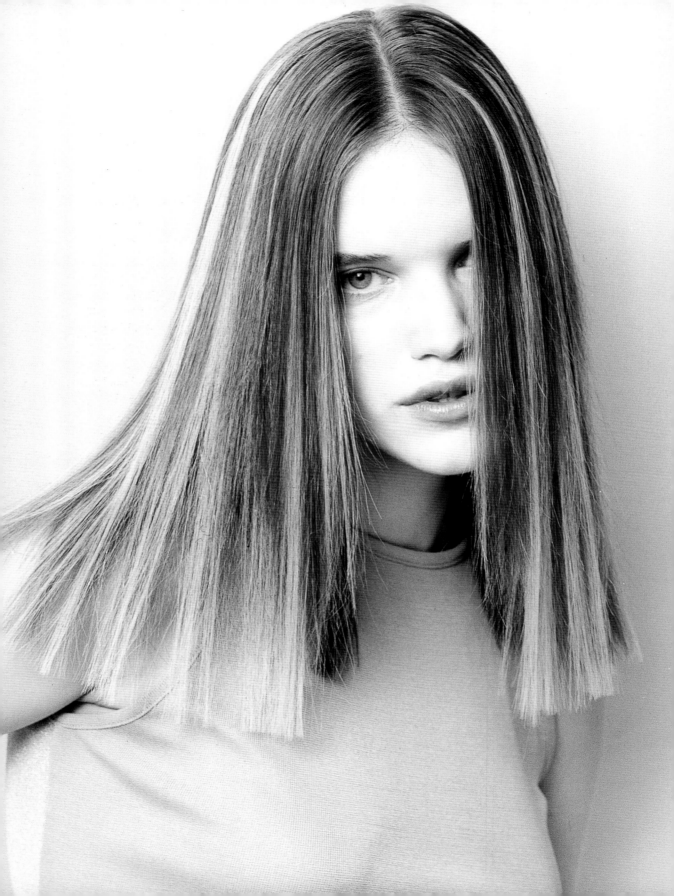

natural grey. Sometimes the natural shade can go yellowish and dull, in which case a rinse that softens the yellow and enhances the silver can work well. It's also important to keep grey hair scrupulously clean and conditioned: grey hair shows up dust and grime easily, and while glossy grey hair has many advantages, dull has none.

If you want to turn your grey hair pink like Zandra Rhodes or purple like Italian *Vogue* style-queen Anna Piaggi, all you need is the confidence to carry it off. This generation of women has decreed that there are no rules about how you should look as you grow older.

While there will always be a small percentage of women who cherish the idea of the bizarre and the different, most women prefer the more natural-looking colour change. Getting that look is now a more sophisticated process than ever. A tint and a bleach can be used on the same head to bring light and shade as well as a sense of movement to the style. So technologically advanced are some of the high-lift tints around that many on the spectrum from blonde to mid-mouse no longer need to bleach their hair. The best combination for a really good blonde effect is fine highlights around the hairline and parting, simulating what the sun does to hair, with heavier, chunkier lights underneath. Or, just for fun, do the reverse. We did this for Julia Carling: she had highlights throughout and then chunks of blonde at the top and the front.

And we've just devised an even subtler method of getting lighter shade at the front and top of the hair. We've called it *smudging*. Kate Moss was one of the first people we used it on. It's a bit like the paint effect of sponging except much softer and more delicate. You smudge a little high-lift tint around the hairline and whoosh it away towards the ends. It's very soft and extremely pretty.

Jemima Khan, who has been a client for a long time, is a great example of the sunkissed look. She has near perfect hair: the texture is neither too fine nor too thick, and you can do almost anything with it. You can leave it straight, wave it or make it curly. It's a dark mouse shade that lends itself easily to colour change. We use a mixture of fine and slightly thicker lights for Jemima, putting the finer ones at the front and top to give her that perfect creamy, buttery, sun-in-the-hair look.

Colouring is a great way to give fine hair some extra body. Mariella Frostrup, another client, has fine, flyaway, Scandinavian hair. When she first came to me she had a one-length bob. To give her hair more body I not only put layers through it but also gave it some extra blonde lights.

While there are no longer any unbendable rules in hair styling and colouring, there are a few guidelines worth noting:

- For a more natural effect, keep within your own colour range. Pale blonde hair rarely works well with olive skin, although that hasn't put off some seriously glamorous Italians like Donatella Versace. If you don't have that sort of confidence, stick to creamier tones with pale highlights and a few lowlights to add depth.

- There are shades of red to suit most people. If you have fair skin you can take anything from a strawberry blonde to the more vibrant reds. Dark and olive skins look best in auburn and burgundy shades. Only avoid red if your complexion tends to the ruddy.

- If you long to go blonde but aren't sure which shade suits you, check the colour of your eyes. If your eyes are green or brown, veer towards golden blonde; if your eyes are grey or blue, veer towards the ash shades.

- For the first-timer or the timid would-be blonde, do it in stages. It's easier to go progressively paler at first and then later gradually introduce darker bits or lowlights.

- If you want to cover up grey hair, ask for highlights or a permanent tint. However, never use a permanent tint more than two shades darker than your natural colour. Only a little darker is needed to cover the grey and also to add depth.

■ As we age, lighter colours are more flattering.

■ If you want to hang on to your grey – and it can look immeasurably chic – also remember that it can look incredibly dull. If it looks dull, it's draining the skin tone too. Highlights or lowlights are a good method of keeping the brightness in by providing a shade between your own colour and the grey.

■ A change of colour often requires a change of make-up too.

■ A change of colour also requires time and commitment. You can't transform the shade of your hair and then leave it: hair grows, colours fade. There's always the question of upkeep. Blondes and highlights are the most demanding and time-consuming, so don't enter into the arrangement unless you're determined to keep it. Blonde hair with dark roots was fashionable when grunge was about but then grunge didn't last long and really only worked on the very young or the very hip such as Courtney Love.

■ Remove the fear factor. Reassure yourself that these days most colour treatments by reputable colourists don't damage the hair in any way. But be kind to colour-treated hair. Look after it, protect it from the sun – however much time and money you've spent chasing the effect sun has on hair! – and always use products specially formulated for chemically coloured hair.

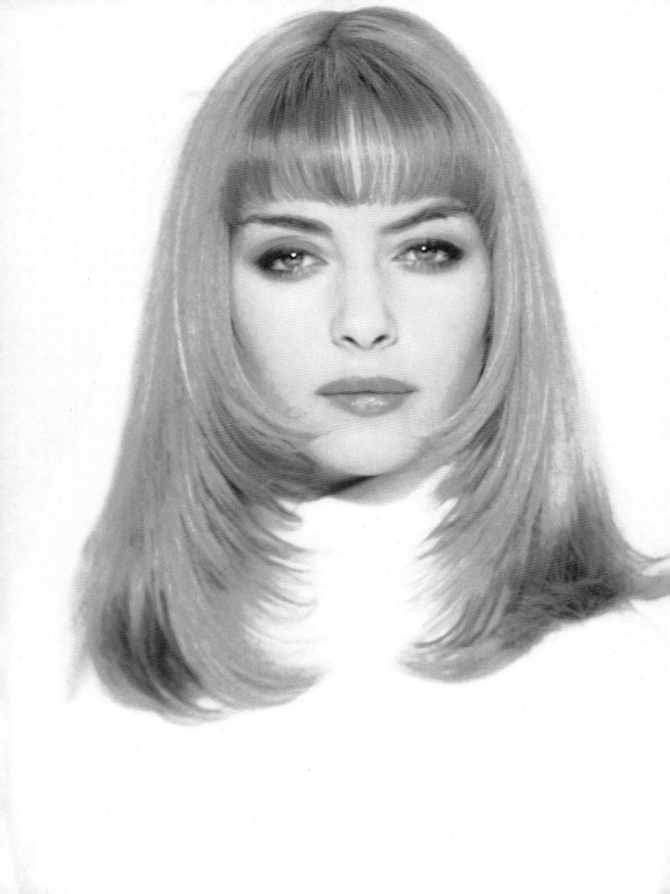

DOING IT FOR YOURSELF

ONE OF THE FASTEST-GROWING MARKETS IN HAIR COLOUR IS FOR TONE-ON-TONE SEMI-PERMANENT COLOURS. NOW IF YOU HAVE MID TO DARK HAIR AND ALL YOU WANT TO DO IS ENRICH THE COLOUR, THEN I'D SAY IT'S FINE TO DO THIS AT HOME. THAT IS, PROVIDED YOU READ THE INSTRUCTIONS. IT'S EXTRAORDINARY HOW MANY PEOPLE STILL READ ONLY HALF THE INSTRUCTIONS, THEN DECIDE THEY KNOW WHAT TO DO, AND WONDER WHAT WENT WRONG LATER WHEN IT SO INEVITABLY DOES. JUST BE CAREFUL IF YOU HAVE A PERM OR ANY HENNA IN YOUR HAIR – EITHER OF THESE MAY CAUSE A REACTION.

BE WARY OF ANY PROCESS THAT REQUIRES THE MIXING OF TWO COMPONENTS TOGETHER. THESE SHOULD BE LEFT TO THE PROFESSIONALS. ANYONE NOT TRAINED AND PRACTISED SHOULD BE WARY OF MIXING AND USING CHEMICALS – FOR THAT'S WHAT THEY ARE.

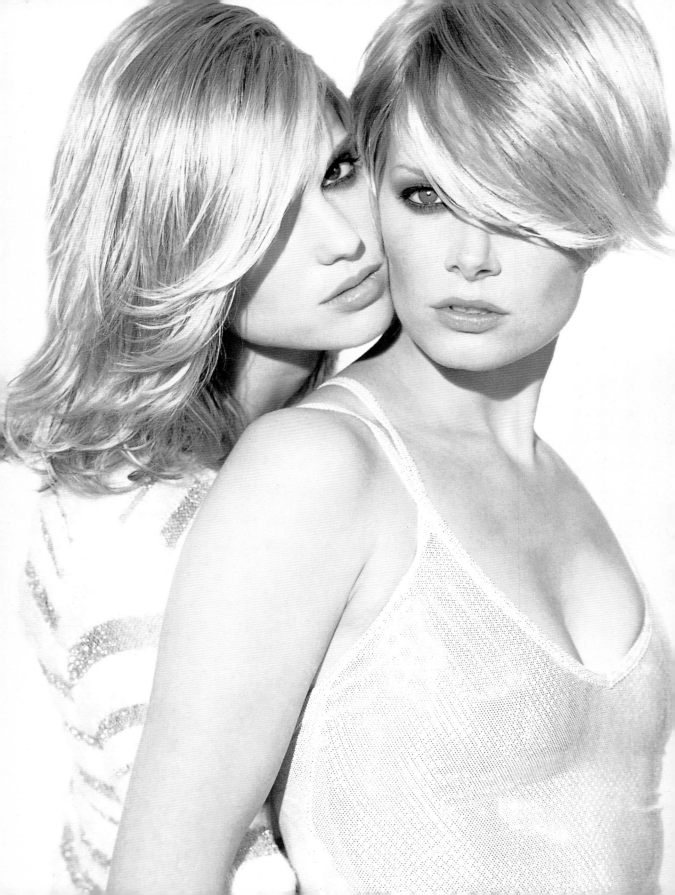

BE BLONDE

h

hair care

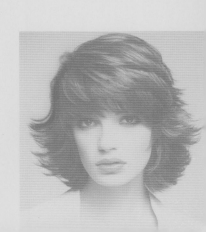

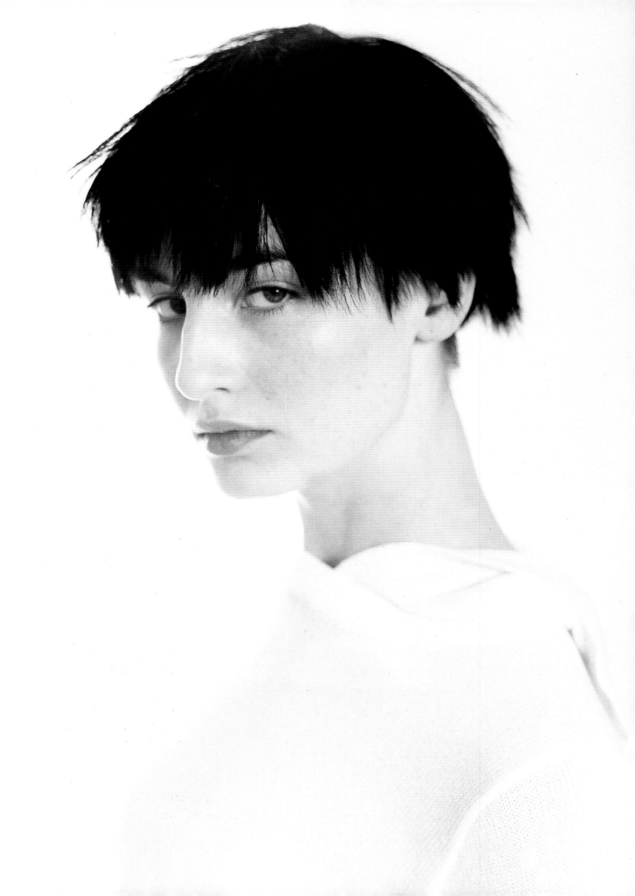

The kind of hair we have is down to our genes, whether it's fine, frizzy, thick, lustrous, wavy or straight. Of course, that doesn't mean you're completely stuck with it, because you can do certain things with most hair. What it does mean is that you need to learn what type of hair you have and understand how to deal with it.

All you need is:

- An understanding of your hair type – and what it can do
- A decent hairdresser – who looks after your hair and shows you how to look after it yourself
- The right equipment – and to know how to use it
- The right products

First, the facts. A strand of hair is composed of a protein known as keratin and grows from a single follicle (sac). Each of us is born with a specific number of follicles in our scalp, a number which doesn't change throughout our life. An average head has between 90,000 and 120,000 follicles. Blondes have more because their hair is fine, while redheads have the least because their hair is thick, which is why it looks so luxuriant. The rest are in between.

Each individual hair has three layers – a transparent inner core known as the medulla, a middle layer called the cortex, which denotes much of the texture and colour, and then the outer layer or cuticle, which consists of overlapping cells, all of them dead. These cells may be dead but they declare to the world the condition of each hair. If they overlap in an orderly fashion like fish scales, then the hair is smooth and reflects the light. If they are damaged, whether from environmental attacks, too much heat from hairdryers or other appliances, or overprocessing of colour or perms, then they won't lie smoothly and reflect the light, and hair looks dull.

For something that's basically dead, hair is remarkably resilient. A strand of hair is stronger than copper wire of the same diameter. Its elasticity is phenomenal: it can stretch to almost 30 per cent of its length. Way below the surface, however, is plenty of life. This is where all the action is taking place. Each hair has its own root (the papilla) and each root is a factory, supplied with nutrients by the blood and kept healthy by the action of nerves and muscles. Although more than a hundred hairs fall out each day, hair continues to grow. Pull a single hair out by its root and you will find a little white blob at the end of it, but inside the scalp the papilla is still intact and works away to produce a new hair. It's pretty reassuring to know that roots are so relentless, that no matter how badly hair is treated it fights back. But this has its downside, surprisingly. It's why women have such a difficult time getting rid of unwanted hair elsewhere on their bodies. Plucking, waxing and depilatories get rid of the hair, but they don't subdue the root.

Obviously, as we get older, regeneration slows down, like in every other cell in the body, but it doesn't stop. From the age of forty-five onwards most people notice a change in hair texture, along with a slight thinning. But even though in older women you see wider partings, most of the hair still grows. This should tell us that it's worth rewarding our hair's resilience with the right treatment, the right diet and the right products. Because if our hair sticks to us through thick and thin (different if you're a man where baldness can be a problem), at least we should learn to care for it properly. It responds amazingly well to kindness and consideration.

The **Nicky Clarke** Five Golden Rules of Hair Care:

- A well-balanced diet – protein with lots of fresh fruit and vegetables
- The right shampoos, conditioners and intensive conditioning treatments for the hair
- Gentle treatment from dryers, brushes, accessories
- A good cut
- If things begin to go wrong, such as excess hair loss or thinning (in a woman), get help instantly, whether from your hairdresser, doctor or a trichologist. Most conditions, if caught early enough, can be dealt with reasonably easily. A responsible hairdresser will advise you if you need to see a doctor: it's in his interests, too, that your hair should look healthy and happy.

Exercise, diet and supplements I've already dealt with, but how about products – how can anybody know which ones to choose? I admit that the choice of shampoos and conditioners is almost limitless these days. Go into any supermarket or high street chemist and the number is overwhelming. I'm surprised anybody has the time, let alone the energy, to work their way through the ranges to find the right one for them. What usually happens is that people find a product they like and stick with it. That's fine up to a point, but hair can change and so can its needs, and you may have to make the adjustments.

Products have stuck to the same system for a long time: they are made for dry, normal and oily hair. But what is 'normal' hair? In this country most people have fine, limp, what I call English-type hair – so that could be regarded as normal. I've spent the last twenty or so years looking at different heads, working with different hair types and I know what people really want:

- People with fine, limp hair want extra body

- People with coarse, frizzy hair want to be able to smooth it down

- Everybody wants shinier hair

And so, in our Hairomatherapy, Sport and Men's ranges, there are products that provide solutions. Lesley and I have always been particularly keen on aromatherapy, not only because so many of the extracts are beneficial to hair upkeep, but also because their scents make them great to use and give hair a fine aroma. There's a Gentle Shine Shampoo, for example. This is fine for everyday use as it's a mild pH-balanced cleanser, and it's got juniper and lime to invigorate the scalp, vitamin E and panthenol to maintain the hair's natural body and shine, along with a fusion of aloe vera, wheatgerm and jojoba, among other plant extracts, to protect and strengthen the hair.

For fine, flyaway hair I'm particularly proud of our Hair Thickening Shampoo. Natural polymers and panthenol work on each individual hair shaft, lifting and thickening even the finest strand. Extracts of spearmint and sea kelp add volume and boost shine.

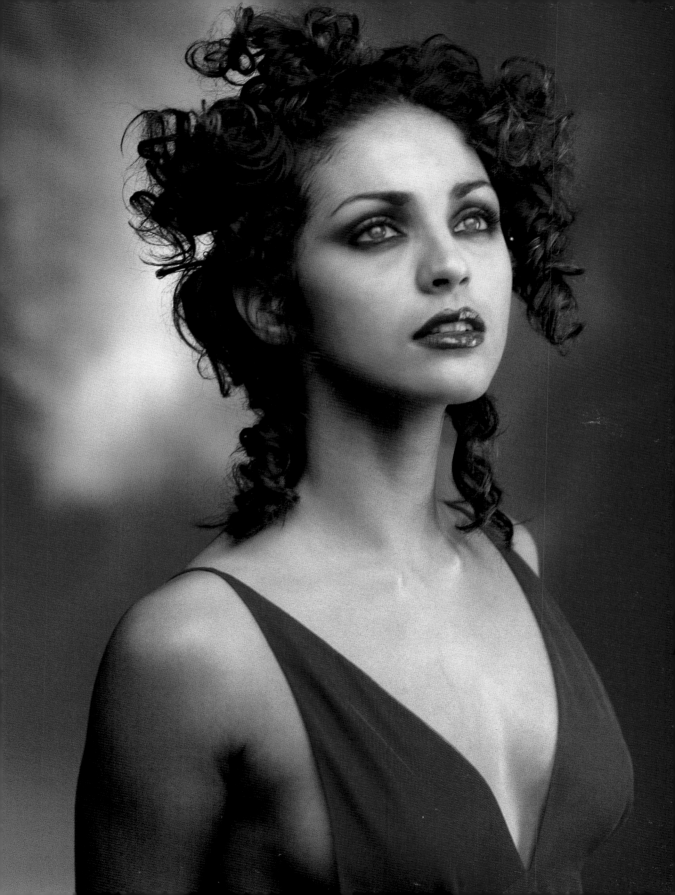

It can take a lot of time, effort and heat to make dry, frizzy hair do what the wearer wants. It's possibly the most difficult of all hair types to live and deal with, and the least likely to reflect shine and depth because of all its frizz and curls. For this hair we've produced Frizz Control Shampoo, an incredible formulation using aloe vera and wheatgerm to seal the cuticle and leave the hair looking silky. It also has extracts of ylang ylang and sage to help relax the hair.

All chemically treated hair has had its structure changed, which can leave it looking dull and lifeless. Our Perm and Colour Therapy Shampoo is devised to redress the imbalance, with sandalwood, hops and wheatgerm among the ingredients that help restore shine and pliability to the hair.

How to shampoo your hair

Considering it is for most of us the first piece of beauty care we learn, it's astonishing how many people still do not know how to shampoo properly.

It's purely a matter of choice how often you shampoo; no frequency is either right or wrong. Clean hair is, of course, the first step to healthy-looking hair and if you live in a town or city you'll find that hair collects dust and dirt faster and quicker than if you live in the country. Many people find they need to shampoo more frequently in hot months than cool or cold ones. But it's down to you.

However often you wash your hair, it is important to do it well. It's possible, otherwise, to damage hair during a perfectly routine hair wash. The first step is to comb through your hair with a wide-toothed comb. This helps loosen particles of dirt or bits of dead skin from the scalp. It also gets rid of tangles, which are easier to get out of dry hair than wet hair. (Remember that hair is at its weakest when wet, making it vulnerable to damage.) A minute or two of gentle scalp massage will also help loosen dust and dirt from the scalp.

Now, using warm water, wet the hair thoroughly. Pour shampoo into the palm of your hand, rub both hands together and then gently stroke it on to your hair. This allows a more even and gentle distribution of shampoo than you get if you pour it straight on to your hair. Be sparing with shampoo: a single dollop the size of a 50-pence piece should be sufficient if you wash daily. If you shampoo every two or three days you may need a little more, along with a second application of shampoo. As you wash your hair, you can give yourself another, easy-going scalp massage, which not only helps cleanse the scalp but invigorates the cells and blood supply.

Now rinse the hair with lots of clean, warm water. A shower spray attachment is the easiest, quickest and best way of rinsing away shampoo – why do you think hairdressers always use one? Just when you think you have rinsed every element of shampoo away and your hair is squeaky clean, give it another go – one of the main reasons why hair can look dull is insufficient rinsing. Now, before you apply conditioner, pat excess moisture out of your hair with a towel.

Apply the conditioner. Most people just need a light coating to help de-tangle the hair and smooth down the cuticles. Most conditioners act immediately, so leaving them on for two or three minutes doesn't necessarily improve their effectiveness. Do as you did with the shampoo: pour a dollop of conditioner into the palm of the hand, rub your hands together and smooth the conditioner over your hair. Don't rub conditioner into the scalp: hair usually needs conditioning along its length, not at the root. Rinse off with meticulous care.

Depending on your hair type and how well or badly you've been treating it, the occasional deep-conditioning treatment will be necessary. I suggest either once a week or once a fortnight for most hair types.

When you've rinsed away the conditioner, wrap the hair in a towel and pat it dry: don't rub it. Leave the towel wrapped around your head for a few minutes to soak up more moisture.

DID

TOO HOT WATER

TOO LITTLE WATER

TOO LITTLE RINSING

TOO MUCH ROUGH HANDLING
AND SUBSEQUENT TANGLING
– NO RUBBING

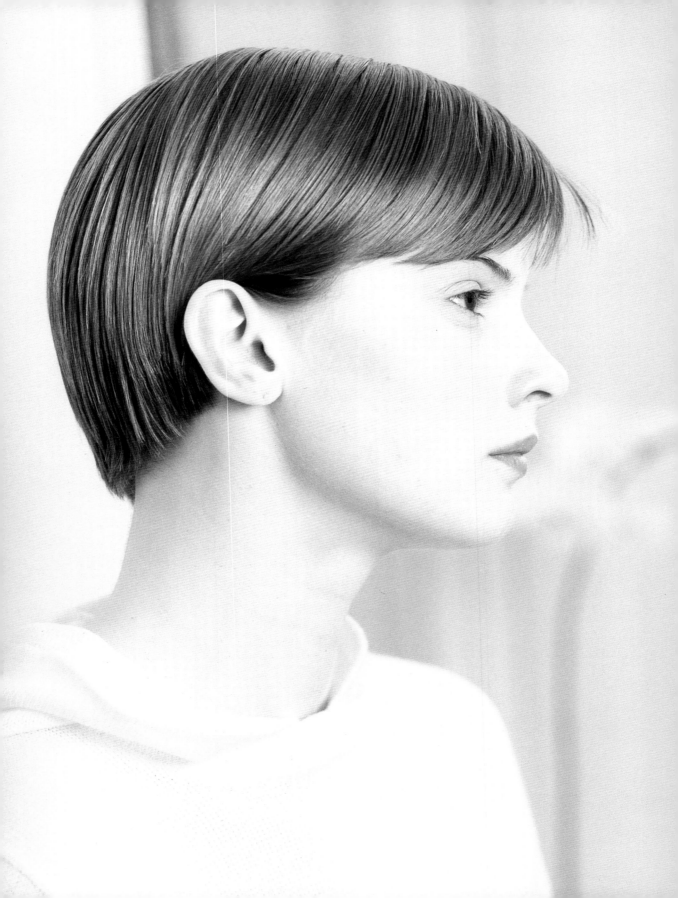

Styling

The type of styling product you use is determined by the type of hair you have and the effect you want to create. I have a full range of products, designed to complement all the other products. I prefer to work with lotions; that way I can position the volume where I need it. I often finish with a lick of wax or serum for a little high definition. Experiment until you find what's right for you: right for your hair type and easy for you to use at home. Here's a glossary guide to each type and what it's good for.

Mousse, the first of the new-generation of gravity-defying products to come on to the market, adds body, volume and hold to most hair types. It's good for fine or short hair which needs lift from the roots, and it also helps to boost curls as well as straighten wavy hair. It's also great for giving added texture to short hair. For most uses take an amount the size of a golf ball and spread it evenly through 80 per cent dry hair (if your hair is curly you can have it slightly wetter when you apply mousse), and then either blow-dry, finger-dry or scrunch.

Volumizing spray is one of the most versatile of all styling products. It's particularly good for when you want to be quite specific about where you add volume. Simply spray on to root area when hair is almost dry. It gives extra body, volume and fullness to hair by coating it, making it thicker and easier to style. Good for all hair types that need root lift, particularly fine, straight and limp hair, and good for all lengths of hair. It's not so good for coarse and wiry hair – for this hair use Frizz Control Conditioning Blow Dry Lotion. The protective elements in this lotion help control frizz and eliminate static while giving wiry hair the extra protection from heat it requires because it takes longer than straight hair to dry.

Gels are good for taming wild hair and giving lasting hold to curls; they also keep fringes and flicks in place. They're not ideal for very fine hair because they can weigh it down. Use on both damp and almost dry hair and then leave to dry naturally, or smooth it on dry hair to control and add shine. Gels are great for a slicked, slightly wet look.

Wax is a great innovation for the Nineties. It should be used sparingly, on dry hair, concentrating on the ends to add gloss definition and shine – as a bonus it helps control static too. It can be used on permed, naturally curly or coarse hair, but not on fine, long hair, which it will make limp. Take a tiny amount, rub it between your palms to warm it then run it through hair for that edgy, modern look. It gives a very polished, groomed effect if used all over the hair, and it is terrific for creating spikes on the ends of short hair.

Serum, the latest favourite product, can be used on dry hair for instant shine or on damp hair for extra shine before styling. Use only a minute amount, otherwise it gets too heavy for the hair. It also helps control static. Healthy hair naturally carries a positive electrical charge, but chemical processing, too much heat or environmental factors such as cold temperatures or walking on nylon carpets can cause hair to take on a negative charge. The hairs repel one another and become flyaway and unmanageable. Fine hair is most vulnerable to static: it has a thin cortex that allows static electricity to build up more easily. My Frizz Control Shine Serum controls and protects even the most unmanageable hair and is great for restraining static, while my Spray-on Serum dispenses a fine mist for a light and even coverage and a great, glossy effect.

Hairspray is the old favourite for holding hairstyles in place and preventing fine hair flopping in damp weather. It's a fixing, not a styling, product. To get the best effects, hold the can about 10 inches away from your hair and spray lightly.

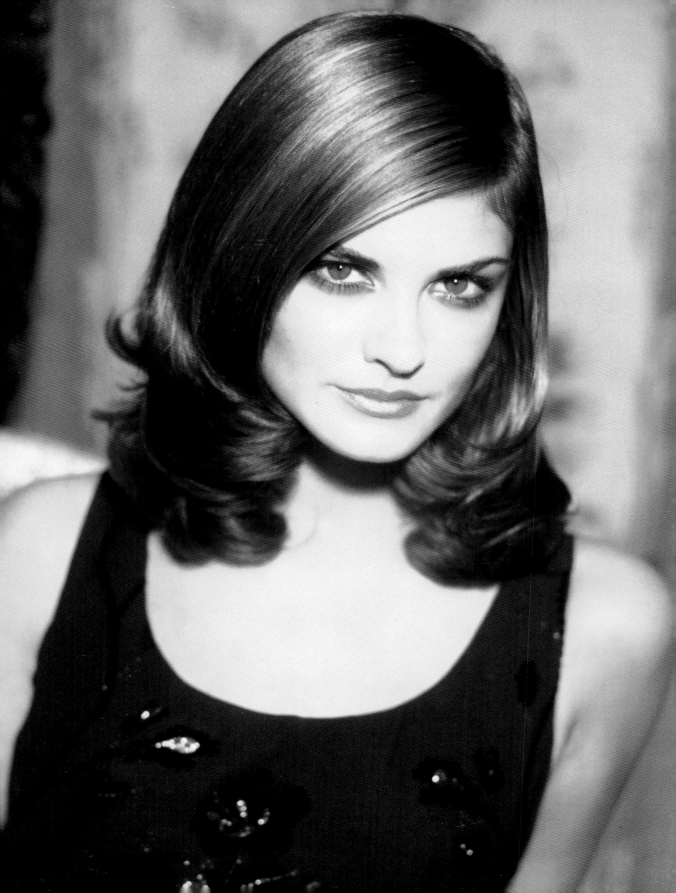

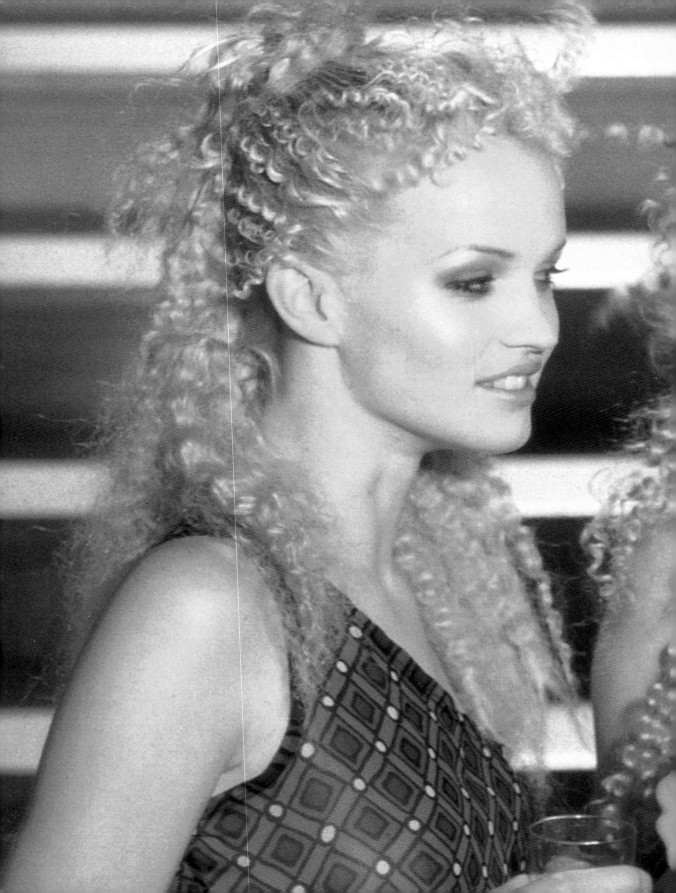

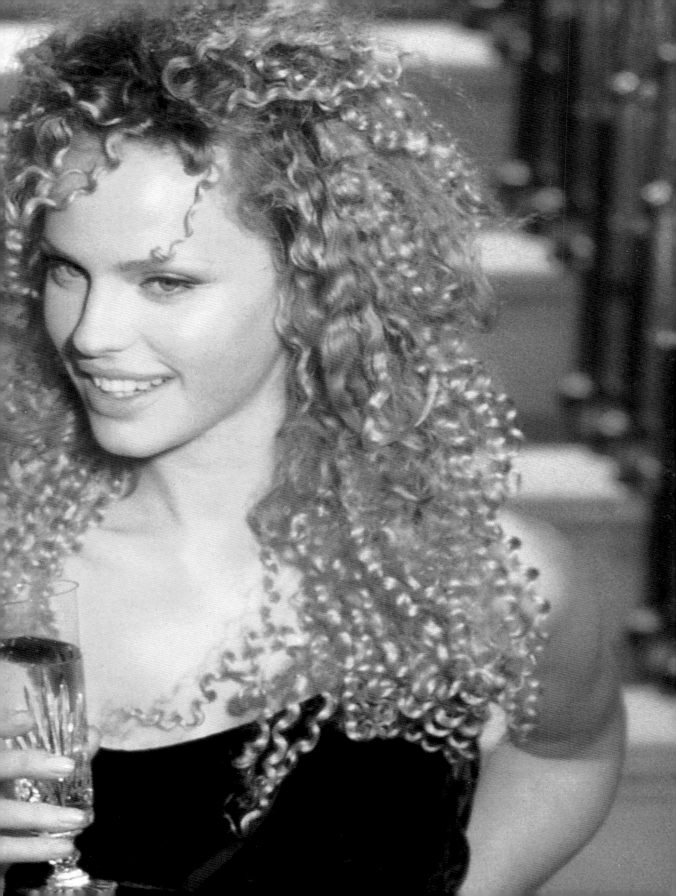

THE BEST WAY TO BLOW-DRY

1 A hairdryer with a minimum strength of 1500 watts, two speeds and two heat settings *plus* a cold button. The cold button is needed right at the end of drying to set the line before removing the brush.

2 The right brushes: most hairstyles probably need at least two. It depends on the length of your hair. With very short hair you can get away with one, but usually you need a large and a medium-sized brush. They should be round and they must be bristle. Hair should not be wrapped around the brush because that leads to tangles, pulling and breakages. The brush should be big enough to get under the hair and lift from the roots. Remember, the tighter you want the curl, the smaller the brush should be. The dryer should run down the hair to keep the cuticles flat.

3 The styling product of your choice: gel, mousse or volumizing spray.

4 A selection of clips and rollers to hold the hair back, give it lift or create pin curls.

Once the tools are assembled, you're ready to dry.

■ First pat excess moisture from your hair with a towel and then go through with a wide-toothed comb. Any tangles should be dealt with from the middle of the shaft to the end – don't pull from the root. Hair loses up to 25 per cent of its elasticity when wet and will eventuallly snap if you pull too hard. Never use a brush on wet hair for the same reason.

■ Start to dry the hair using the hairdryer on a warm setting. Occasionally ruffle the hair close to the roots with your fingers, and to get extra lift hold your head upside down and direct air at the roots.

■ Unless you have really curly or frizzy hair, get the hair almost 80 per cent dry, and then apply your styling product. Up until then, if you try to do too much you'll flatten it. This may seem strange but trust all my years of working with different types of hair. When people first see me work they cannot believe how dry I like the hair to be. I even do most of my cutting when the hair is 80 per cent dry. I do the rough cut when the hair is wet to give me the blueprint, the line of the shape, but only as it dries can I see how it moves and falls. When the hair is almost dry, I cut in the finer details and refine as I go. If you get the cut right and it looks OK at that just-dry stage, then the rest is easy. The same applies to styling.

■ Section off the important areas, namely the top, front and sides, and concentrate on that. As you dry and smooth each section, put it on a Velcro roller to maintain its lift and volume while you gradually work your way down each side from the crown.

■ Once you've got the top sorted out you can concentrate on the back.

■ When your hair is completely dry, unwind the rollers and go through the hair loosely using either your fingers or a comb.

■ Now is the time to make adjustments. Extra definition can be given to waves, curls or strands with a spot of wax, and everything can be kept in place with a quick squirt of hairspray.

■ If your hair looks much better once it's had a few rollers in, it might be worth investing in a portable hood-style dryer – you only need keep it on for ten minutes.

- Dryers with diffuser attachments are the gentlest way of drying exceptionally curly and wavy hair. They are also great for encouraging any curl you have in your hair.

- Styling depends a lot on the wrist action – a bit like playing squash – so try to switch the dryer from hand to hand to get a more symmetrical drying pattern. Few of us are naturally ambidextrous, but after a bit of practice the technique gets easier.

The most important thing that styling products can do is what they are meant to do. Too many products on the market are almost afraid to work. If you use dollops of mousse the size of a grapefruit then the mousse is not worth having. Indeed, it's going to make the hair feel like candyfloss.

I wanted my products to work perfectly, and I needed them to work in a professional capacity too. (I'm always amazed when salons who have their own lines use other manufacturers' products for 'professional use'.) I use my products all the time in my salon. That's my guarantee that they work well.

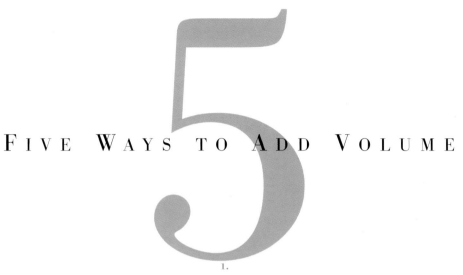

FIVE WAYS TO ADD VOLUME

1.

Use volumizing sprays and mousses.

2.

Turn your head upside down to blow-dry the roots and help lift the hair – if you have short hair all you might need after this is simply to smooth the ends over with a brush.

3.

Add a diffuser attachment to your dryer and move it in circles to separate the roots.

4.

For styling longer hair, divide it into sections and blow-dry each section in the opposite direction to the way it will naturally fall. This means you're blowing the sides upwards towards the top of your head and blowing the back forwards.

5.

When the hair is dry, gently backcomb to add more body and fullness.

TO PERM OR NOT TO PERM

Any number of different names are given to perms, but in most cases the process is the same and in essence has not changed since the very first one was introduced, although ingredients and procedures have become gentler and more sophisticated.

A perm changes the structure of the hair. To change the shape of the hair each shaft has to be deconstructed and softened chemically. A perming solution is applied to the hair, which is then wound round a roller or curler. The size of the curler determines the strength of the curl: larger curler = softer curl. The chemical softens the structure of the hair, which is then bent to take on the shape of the curler. When the desired amount of curl has been achieved, a neutralizing agent is used to harden the hair and fix the curl. The same process is used for straightening hair, the only difference being that the hair is combed straight from the roots until it softens sufficiently to retain the required straightness.

THESE ARE THE TYPES OF PERM AVAILABLE:

Root perms, where the chemical is applied only to the roots to add body and lift to lank hair. This process needs to be done very carefully to avoid damaging the scalp.

Spot perms provide root lift, bounce and shape to flat areas such as crowns and sides or to limp fringes.

Body waves are a much gentler approach, using large rollers to give volume and lift. Body waves don't last as long as a normal perm.

Weave perms adds texture and body. The hair is sectioned and not all sections are permed.

Spiral perms are the fiercest of all and should only be done if hair is strong and in tip-top condition. The hair is twisted before being wound on to rollers to give a sort of pre-Raphaelite effect.

Perming is less popular now that there are so many products that can give hair extra body. If you want a perm, make sure you go to a reputable salon. I cannot say this often enough – anything that involves chemicals and especially the mixing and combining of chemicals should really be done by experts.

PERMING TIPS

- Always make sure hair is in tip-top condition before having a perm. Lavish lots of extra care on it for two or three weeks beforehand, giving it deep-conditioning treatments to make sure it retains all its moisture. Remember to continue afterwards with lots of care and attention.

- Leave at least a week, and preferably two, between perming and colouring your hair – otherwise you could end up with hair like straw.

- As your hair grows, the perm will gradually drop from the root. This is when you need to decide whether to have a root perm, a spot perm or to wait and have a full perm once you can trim the gradually weakening ends. Never be tempted to apply one perm on top of another – it will weaken and eventually destroy your hair.

- Most perms add volume, bounce and style to flat, lank and limp hair. Just treat them with respect.

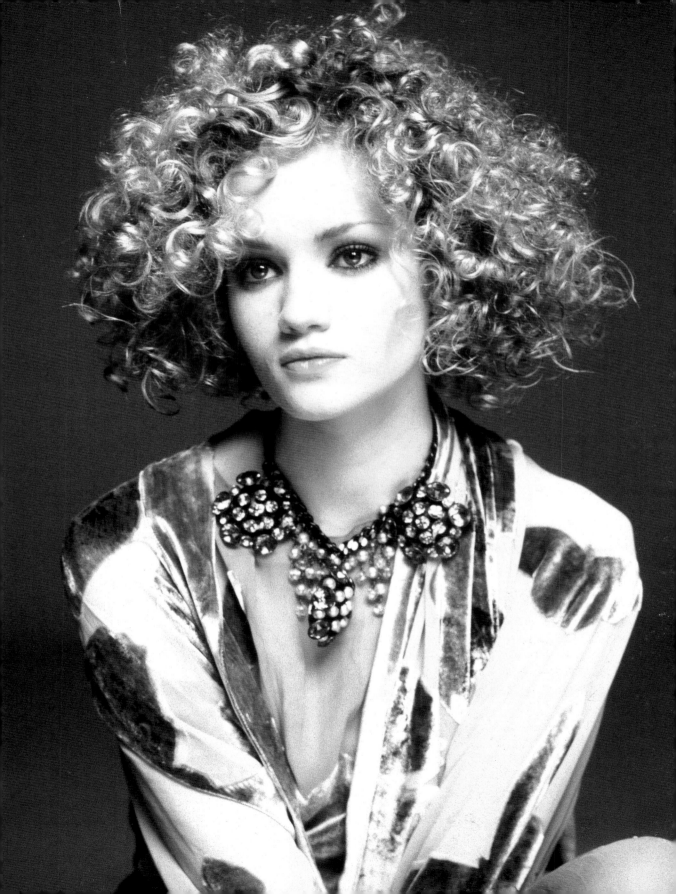

The Fabulous Forties and Beyond

The babyboomers, those who were teenagers in the late Sixties, have absolutely no intention of ageing like their mothers. They have been in the vanguard of the changing lives and looks of women for the last thirty years and they're not going to lie down quietly in their forties, fifties and sixties. But neither do they want to hang on to the looks they had way back when – they know there's nothing more ageing than a look that's past its sell-by date, not to mention its prime. That's not to say you won't see the odd example of the baby-doll long, straight hair of the late Sixties, or the bubble perm of the Seventies, or a drooping Farrah Fawcett (she gave that up herself over a decade ago).

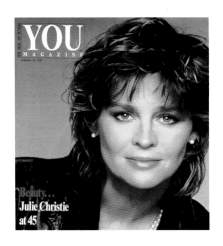

Actress Julie Christie came to London for this shoot from her home in Wales, complete with a badly grown-out perm. We decided to go for the chop, and she ended up looking great.

Only recently Cher complained about how awful being fifty is. She has great bones, wonderful eyes and a great figure – but she'd look a whole lot better if she got a new hairstyle. She might even enjoy being fifty. Goldie Hawn has never let age bother her, and while her style has remained very similar she's adapted its shape and colour as she's got older. Catherine Deneuve is a woman who could almost be said to have invented style. I know she once said that after the age of forty a woman has to choose between her face or her body, but both of hers still look in great shape and her hairstyle – short and elegant – is terrific.

Julie Christie's in her fifties and looks better than ever. She's shown how to adapt and change as you get older. And Joan Collins, who last year picked up her bus pass, has never looked anything other than ultra-glamorous. Neither tries to look young; both try and succeed at looking terrific. Age is something that happens to us all. We might as well get to grips with it and live it the way we want with the looks we want.

Madonna, for heaven's sake, is now forty. Now *there's a woman whose hair I would really love to do*. But mostly I'd just love to meet her – there's probably very little I could do with her hair that would impress or improve her. This is a woman who has had some of the best hairstyles and used some of the best hairdressers in the world. She's had every look – her showmanship is amazing. She's had short, long, mid, straight and curly hair, and she's been every colour from black to red to blonde, and occasionally a mixture. And every single style has worked because her attention to detail is second to none.

Madonna and the other style icons can't halt the ageing process, but you can bet anything you like they'll give it a good run for its money. It's a fact of life that as hair gets older it gets thinner: each individual hair gets thinner in diameter and the regenerative process slows up so that each hair takes longer to grow. Your natural colour fades and grey hairs begin to appear.

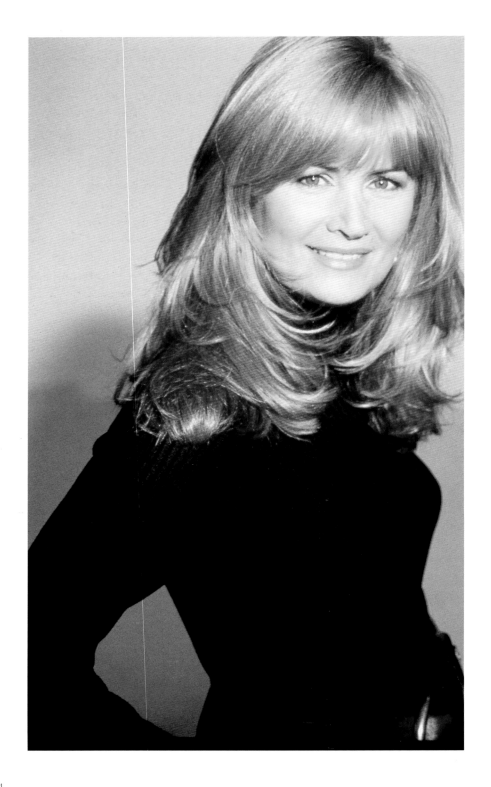

I've already shown you, in Chapter 7, that you can do a lot to maintain hair colour and shade. All you need to be aware of is that hair colour needs to be a little more subtle and have a little more depth as you age, simply to flatter older skin tones. What's really important is to maintain the health and condition of your hair as you get older. A healthy diet is an absolute must, as are certain dietary supplements such as vitamins A, B complex and C, alongside Omega 3 and selenium. Also make sure that you keep your body hydrated with a minimum of eight glasses of water a day.

It's also a good idea to keep the scalp in tip-top condition with a regular massage. This boosts the blood vessels carrying oxygen and essential nutrients to the hair follicles, which will help in regeneration and hair growth. Using the tips of the fingers in small rotating movements on the scalp, move from the front and sides on to the crown and back. Do this for two or three minutes every day. Then take bunches of hair, hold halfway down the length and pull them upwards until you feel the scalp tingle. Do this for two or three minutes every day and your hair will reap the benefits. Be sure, though, never to rub the scalp – this will irritate it.

Remember that one of the great assets of ageing is the innate confidence and sense of power it brings. No one knows this better than today's women, which is why there are so few rules as to how they should look. In their mothers' day a woman hit forty, got a nice perm and kept her hair short and her clothes sensible for the rest of her life. Their daughters decided this was not for them. If they want short and spiky they'll have it – as does Zandra Rhodes, and it's pink to boot. If they want tumbling curls like Jerry Hall they go for them. If they want a traditional bob like Anna Ford they'll have that instead.

Even better, they know that modern technology is on their side. They no longer have to put up with dull, thinning hair when there are volumizers, spray-on shines, mousses and gels to help them have lustrous hair for as long as they desire. And should they want purple streaks they can have those too – with the very latest cosmetic, hair mascara. All they need is a hairstylist who moves at the same pace as they do, who will constantly help update and look after their hair.

My wife, Lesley, looks fabulous in her forties.

Couture
Hair

I try to give all my clients couture hair. People ask me how can I justify my prices. They've been saying that ever since I charged £60. Now a first appointment and styling costs £300. But the people who ask these questions are slightly missing the point. I've been a hairdresser for more than twenty years and in that time I've never stopped learning and never stopped refining what I do. Nobody queries what a beautifully made pair of shoes costs, or how much a qualified carpenter costs, but when it's a haircut some people get an attack of moral outrage. We opened our salon in the middle of the last recession and that brought home to me how people will never give up the essentials. They may not have the money to buy another Chanel suit or Versace frock but they still want a decent haircut. And it is this, alongside clear skin and sparkling eyes and teeth, that is fundamental to style and looks. I'm being neither boastful nor bashful when I say that what I do for hair is the equivalent of what a couturier does for clothes – and nobody wears their couture outfit every day like you do your hair. I know what I can do for each individual client, and I know they consider it worth paying for. They are prepared to wait months for a haircut, and in some instances fly halfway around the world a couple of times a year in order to get their hair done by me.

A good hairstyle – one that suits you, your lifestyle and your hair type – is one of the best investments you can make. It's how you face the world, it's what gives you confidence and it can make you look younger and more glamorous. It's like a facelift without the surgery. Better still, if it's well done you can easily look after it yourself at home, while you get on with your life. That's why my styles – the styles I produce and the styles I like – have this casual look and finish, for the days of the rigid 'do' are well and truly gone.

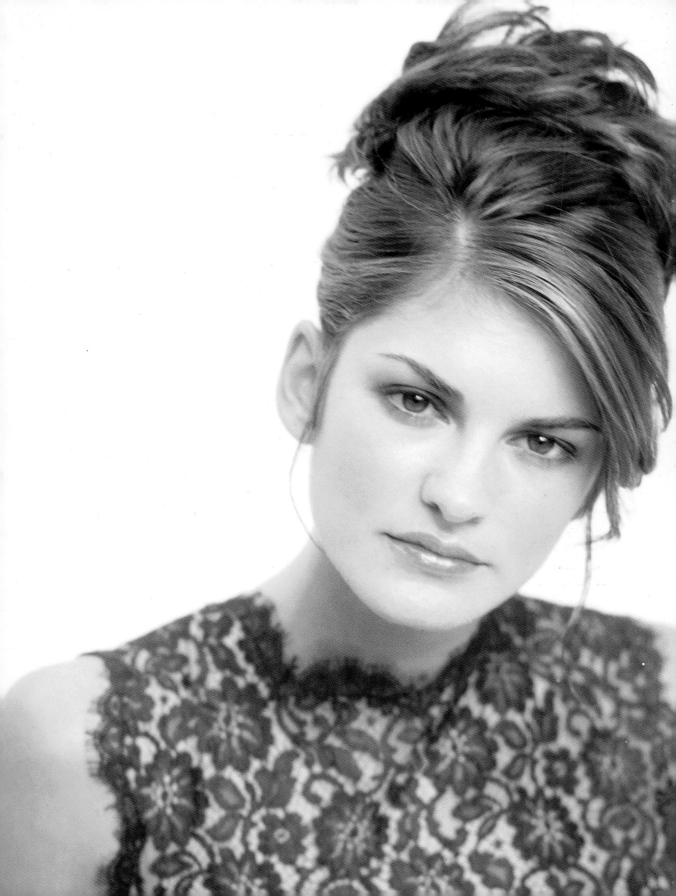

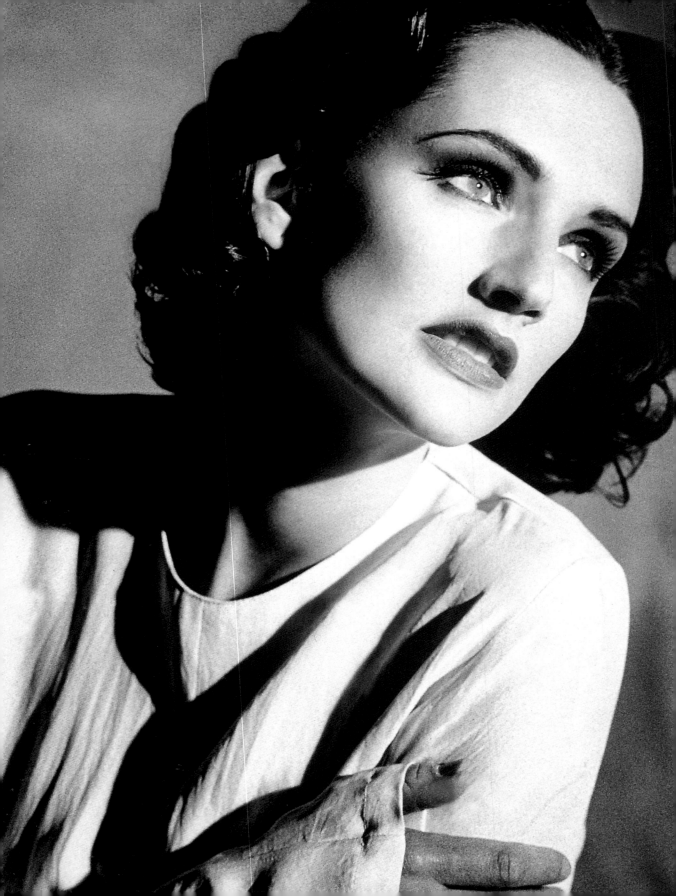

Women are freer now than they have ever been, and their attitudes have changed accordingly. Restrictions in any form are not what they want. Even for formal occasions I always make a style that's softer and consequently more modern and flattering. And I always make sure the style is adapted to suit each person exactly.

There was a time – it may still go on in some salons – when if a stylist or a salon got known for a particular style or cut, that's what the customer got whether it suited her or not. That's OK if that's why the woman went there in the first place. But I cannot work like that. I have to make things work for the individual. That's why I call my styling *couture hair*. A fashion designer will adapt a customer's chosen outfit for her, taking into account the size of her hips, the length of her back, the proportion of her legs. She gets the style she wanted, but it's adapted for her. In the same way, if someone asks me for a style like Anthea's or Selina's, I'll adapt that cut to suit them. Their hair may be a different texture or grow in a different way, their face shape may be different and they may be younger or older. But both the client and I know what she is looking for and I will adapt the style to suit, taking into account the individualities of the person and her hair. That's couture. And that's what my clients like – they don't want to be a carbon copy, but they want the shape and they want it personalized. They also want it updated so that it's fashionable and it suits them. These are women who are neither hair nor fashion victims.

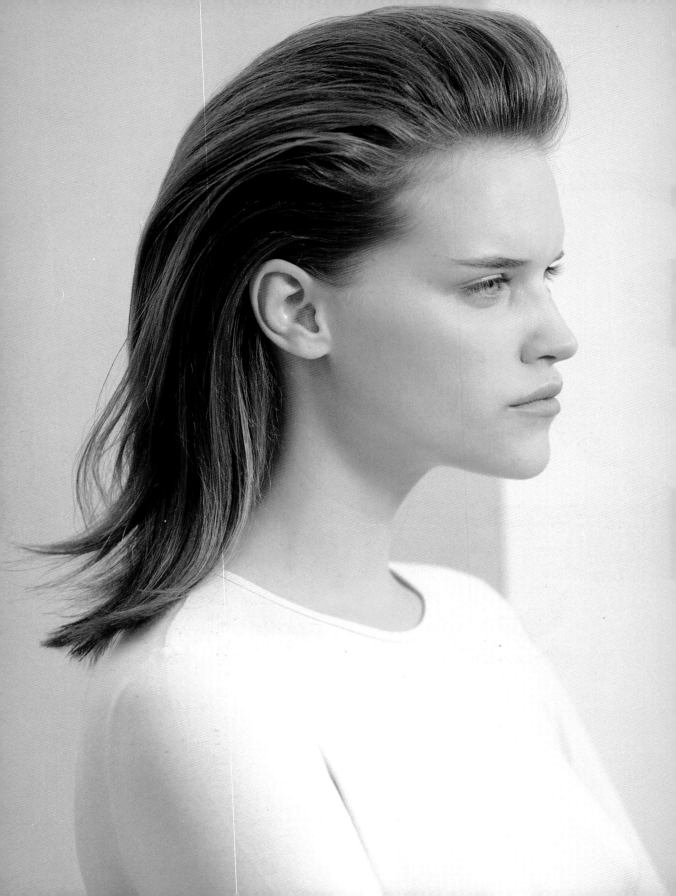

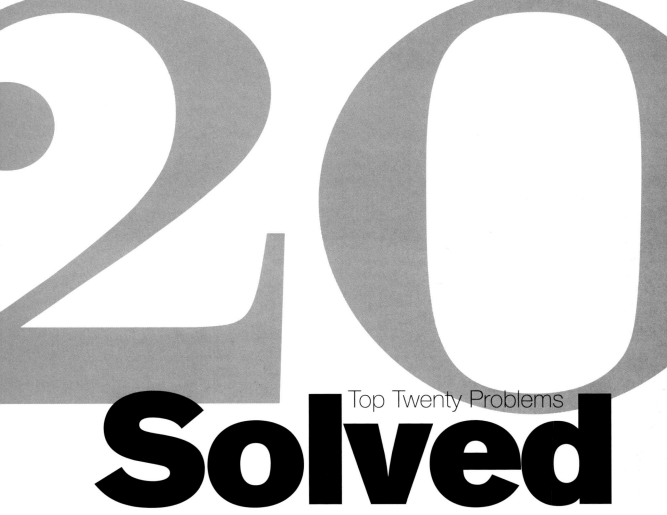

20

Top Twenty Problems
Solved

These are the questions I am most often asked, both in the salon and on my regular TV slot on *This Morning*.

1. Q. I'm never quite sure what my hair's real texture is. How can I find out?

    A. *All you need to do is take a strand of hair, either plucked from your head or unravelled from your hairbrush, and try to break it. If it snaps easily then it's fine in texture, if it breaks only with a bit of effort it's medium, and if it's almost impossible to break then it's coarse.*

2. Q. Why is my hair lank and lifeless, and what can I do about it?

    A. *First check your scalp to see how oily it is. Make a parting down the centre of your hair and gently rub your forefinger back and forth along the parting. Now rub your thumb and forefinger together – if this feels slippery you have an oily scalp. Now you need to find a shampoo that controls the oil, such as my Gentle Shine Shampoo, whose extracts of juniper and lime are useful in oil-control. For styling, use mousse: it has a slightly more drying effect than a spray.*

    Examine your diet – too many processed foods, fried foods and dairy foods contribute to lank hair. Up your intake of fresh fruit and vegetables and drink lots of water. Some prescription drugs – including oral contraceptives – can affect your scalp and hair, so it might be worth checking with your doctor to see if you need to change brands.

    Finally, try to keep your hands away from your hair. The more you fiddle with it the flatter it will lie on your head, and you can also transfer oil to it from your hands.

3. Q. My hair is thick and curly and consequently always goes frizzy. I thought having a short style would help but it doesn't appear to. What can I do about it?

    A. *Curly and frizzy hair is easier to cope with if it's short and you want to keep it curly. But the first rule is not to handle it too much, especially when wet, because that will only increase the frizz. First, however, use a frizz-control shampoo. Ours has plant extracts that help seal the cuticle, enabling the scales to lie flatter. Use this in conjunction with Hairomatherapy's Frizz Control Moisture Balm, and when you have rinsed that out blot hair with a towel: never rub. Dry with a diffuser attachment or simply comb into shape and dry naturally. For a smoother look, style with a round bristle brush and finish with a couple of drops of Frizz Control Shine Serum for long-lasting smoothness. The serum helps prevent moisture loss, acts as a sunscreen and helps stop hair from frizzing in damp air. You can use it between shampoos too.*

4.   Q. What's the best way to straighten my Afro hair?

   A. *To do it yourself with brushes, rollers and electric straightening plates is time-consuming and can be damaging. Much better to put yourself in the hands of the experts and go for a chemical straightening. This is like a perm in reverse: the perming solution is applied to hair that is combed out straight from the roots rather than to hair wrapped in curlers. This helps to soften the hair. As the straightness takes, a neutralizing agent is applied. This is a much trickier process than perming as the hair has to be pulled straight and that can potentially damage the roots – hence the need to get a hairdresser to do it. Use a deep conditioner once or twice a week to help keep hair feeling and looking good.*

5.   Q. Why do I always get a slight kink at the end of my hair when I've used heated rollers or curling tongs?

   A. *Easy – you haven't made sure that the ends are tucked in properly. Always roll the ends under carefully on rollers and tuck them in on properly tongs. You may also be trying to put too much hair in for each curl.*

6.   Q. I think my hairdresser is bored with me – he never really tries to do anything different and seems not to notice how I look. What should I do?

   A. *Before you do anything, tell him what you feel. Perhaps you're so used to each other that, like in many relationships, you've stopped talking. If after this you feel he hasn't responded to your problem – find another stylist. See Chapter 2, Confidence, to help you find one that's right for you.*

7.   Q. I've noticed powdery white flakes on my shoulders – does that mean I have dandruff? How did I get it and what can I do about it?

   A. *It could be that you're suffering from a dry scalp. Turn your head upside down and brush your hair over some dark fabric or paper. If the flakes are small and powdery, it's likely you have a dry scalp. If they are large, clumpy and moist, it's likely you have dandruff. Both can be treated and are temporary conditions. A dry scalp may be caused by stress, tiredness or insufficient rinsing of shampoos and conditioners. Give your scalp a gentle massage once a week with warm oils, such as almond, before shampooing out. Keep hair scrupulously clean, washing frequently with a gentle shampoo.*

   Although dandruff also results in flakes from the scalp, it's more likely to be caused by oily conditions than dry ones. The dead cells from the scalp pick up excess sebum, which is why they can fall in clumps. Use a specially formulated shampoo − there are a number of them on the market − and use it regularly, alternating it with your usual shampoo. We have devised a good anti-dandruff shampoo for our men's range − simply because men tend to suffer from the condition more than women do. Watch your diet too − eat lots of fresh fruit and vegetables and cut down on fats. Try to get regular exercise because it helps send oxygen through the body to regenerate the cells. If the condition persists, see your doctor or consult a trichologist. Don't worry unduly about it: worrying only makes the condition worse. After all, we all come across it at some point in our lives.

8. Q. I want to change the colour of my hair but I hate how roots look − is there anything that can make them less noticeable?

    A *The first thing is to steer clear of any dramatic colour change. Opt for a semi-permanent tint that will fade without leaving noticeable roots. If you have a permanent colour put in, stay within two shades of your natural shade to minimize the demarcation line. Or go for highlights or lowlights. The subtler they are, the more they look as if they have been caused by the sun, and they will often grow out gracefully.*

9. Q. I'd love to have long hair but my hair stops at a certain length and looks raggedy and wispy. Is there anything I can do?

    A. *It sounds to me as if your hair is very thin in diameter, which means it will probably never grow very long. You may never have hair way past your shoulders, but a good and clever cut with layers and movement can give the impression of much longer and fuller hair, as will a soft fringe or graduated layers around the sides. Talk to your hairdresser about aiming for such a cut. Incidentally, different types of hair grow at different rates, although the average is about half an inch a month.*

10. Q. My hair goes through phases of being greasy but recently I was told that even when it's like that I should use a conditioner. Is this true?

    A. *Yes. A conditioner is for your hair and not your scalp, so make sure to apply it along the hair shaft rather than over the scalp area. A conditioner's main job is to flatten the cuticle scales to keep the hair shiny and tangle-free. The last thing your hair needs if it is going through an oily phase is to have tangles combed out, pulling at roots and adding pressure to your scalp. You should also try to establish if there's a pattern to your hair's oily phases − for example, whether it's hormonal, or caused by bad eating. That way you can deal with it much more easily. My light anti-static conditioner is formulated exactly for this type of hair.*

11. Q. I've been told that all-in-one shampoos and conditioners are bad for hair – is this true?

A. *No. Anything that cleans and conditions your hair cannot be bad. These products are terrific for taking to the gym or on holiday or whenever you don't want to be laden down with bottles. They're also good if you're in a hurry, and particularly popular with men. They wouldn't enjoy the success they've had if they didn't work. The formulation allows the conditioner to be held in tiny molecules until the residue of shampoo is rinsed away, when the conditioning particles are then released.*

12. Q. I've just turned forty and my hair seems to be a lot thinner than it used to be, with more coming out on my hairbrush and clothes each day – is it my age?

A. *Age does come into it. By the time we reach fifty, the regeneration of any cell growth has started to slow down. However, there are four other main causes of hair loss in women. Poor nutrition is the cause in 30 per cent of cases. So look to your diet, make sure you have regular meals and don't miss out on protein and iron. In 10 per cent of cases of women under fifty, and 25 per cent of those over fifty, there's a genetic imbalance. A thyroid imbalance is the third possibility but this affects only a small number of women. The fourth possibility is the rare (in women) alopecia areata. If you're seriously worried, consult your doctor and ask him to refer you to a trichologist.*

However, natural causes – ageing and a change in the balance of hormones – are the most likely. Look after your hair with regular washing and conditioning. If it looks better you'll feel better about it. Colour it with highlights, lowlights or semi-permanent tints, because colour helps swell the hair and can make it look more luxuriant. Finally, use volumizers and gels that contain polymers. Almost all of my styling products do. The heat from the dryer swells the polymers, which cling to each shaft of hair, making it appear thicker.

13. Q. Does it really matter which type of brush and comb I use?

A. *Absolutely. Look at what your hairdresser uses and take that as a guideline. I recommend only wide-toothed combs for general use (though the fine-toothed combs are useful for backcombing), as well as for styling any type of hair that needs lifting at the roots, along with coarse curly hair and Afro hair. Brushes must always be boar's bristle: they are gentle and don't scratch or damage the scalp. As with most things, you pays your money and you takes your choice. Cheap plastic brushes are not worth putting anywhere near your hair. They do not have the same smoothing, shine and styling qualities as the bristle variety. And do remember to wash combs and brushes regularly.*

14. Q. I have slightly curly hair and my hairdresser told me that scrunch drying
would help give the curls a lift. How do you do it?

A. *If a hairdresser offers advice such as this, you should always ask him or her to
explain exactly what is meant – most would be only too pleased to tell you. If
you have a diffuser on your hairdryer, let your hair fall into the diffuser bowl
so that its prongs can gently ruffle it. Section it first, then take a handful of
hair and squeeze and push it towards the roots in a concertina way – not too
much hair and not too tightly – as you dry it. Hold for a second or two when
it's dry, or give your hair a blast of cold air from the dryer. Then rub a tiny
amount of serum or wax between your palms and tweak it into the curls to
help separate them and add definition.*

15. Q. Does diet really make a difference to how your hair looks?

A. *Yes, yes and yes. See Chapter 4, which discusses diet and supplements. Your
hair reflects what your health is like. That's why people who've been seriously
ill have dull, lifeless hair. People suffering from eating disorders such as bulimia
and anorexia often have lank, thin hair, and even prescribed drugs can have
an effect on how your hair looks.*

16. Q. I've just had my hair cut and I hate it. What can I do?

A. *Ask yourself why you hate it. Is it because it's too drastic a change and you're
not used to it, or is it that you don't know how to manage it? Whatever the
reason, go back to the hairdresser's and say what you feel. You may just need
the hairdresser to go through all the reasons you chose this style again to
revive your confidence in it. Also ask him or her to show you the easiest way to
style it and look after it. If after all that you still can't stand it, take a deep
breath and remember it's already started growing again. That's the great thing
about hair. Remember, if you don't mind going even shorter, you can still
change your hair quite a lot.*

17. Q. I've noticed more and more hairdressers are offering a scalp massage. What
are the benefits and can I do it myself?

A. *Not only is it a wonderful relaxant, massage also helps stimulate blood supply
to the head, which brings with it all the nutrients and oxygen you need to
encourage healthy hair growth. It's easy to do it yourself. Use fingertips, don't
scratch the scalp and don't rub hair against your scalp either because this can
cause friction and hair breakages. You just need gentle, small rotating
movements. Start at the front, then move to the sides before going on to the
crown and then the back of your head. You need spend no more than a minute
on each section.*

18. Q. Everybody told me my hair would be thick and shiny when I got pregnant but it's quite the opposite – thin and lank. What can I do?

A. *There are some very lucky women whose hair and skin bloom during pregnancy, but this doesn't happen to everyone. Hair mostly doesn't change until after the baby is born. If your hair is really thin, it may be a dietary problem. Consult your doctor, but meanwhile help it to look its best with regular shampooing and conditioning. Soon it will be back to normal.*

19. Q. I coloured my hair myself and it's much darker than I expected it to be. What can I do?

A. *The first thing you can do is nothing. If it's a semi-permanent colour it will fade with time and shampooings. If you've used a permanent colour product, go to your hairdresser – never be tempted to rectify any colour mistake yourself.*

Manufacturers tell us that most problems with home hair colourants arise because people don't read and follow the instructions completely. If you want to DIY, remember to read the instructions to the last letter.

20. Q. I've been brushing my hair twice a day since I was a child and now my hairdresser has told me it's completely the wrong thing to do. Is it?

A. *Too much brushing can cause static on fine hair. In general, if you're careful about the tools you use, it shouldn't harm your hair. A wide-toothed comb is better at freeing dust and dirt particles and is much gentler than a brush. Brushes are best kept for styling.*

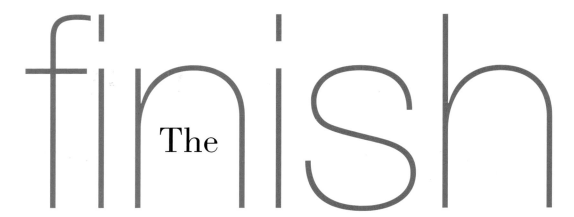

The finish

I take great care over the finish of a style. The finish is an accumulation of a few fine details that take a style from being just OK to terrific. Most of us know someone who on her way out of the hairdressers stopped in the loo to brush through her newly done hair so that it didn't look too set. My finish always helps a style look more natural.

When I'm cutting and styling I never take my eyes off the hair. I look at the way it moves, sits and settles once the air of the dryer is taken away. I swing around in my wheeled chair looking at the style from all sides. This allows me to look at the hair from all angles and from the same level as the client. There's no point standing over a head because that way you only see what it looks like and how it sits from above.

Because I want my styles to look real as opposed to 'done', I do most of my cutting when the hair is almost dry, as I've already explained. That way I know how its movement affects its shape and vice versa. And I never stop refining it until all three elements – shape, style and swing – work as one. Then the hair is blow-dried into the style and finished with the tiny touches that make it both individual and natural: is there enough body in the right places, does it need a tiny touch or tweak to give added definition to a curl or a wave, does it have enough shine to make it look fresh and healthy? It's attention to detail – that's what I like to do.

I want people to be happy with their hair, know that they have a great cut and then forget about it. That's the real power of good hair – and good hairdressing.

Acknowledgements

My family – especially my mum and dad, Lesley and my children.
My incredible, loyal staff – in the salon and the Nicky Clarke hair
care division. Jo Foley for helping me get the words in the right order.
The team at Transworld for their enormous help in realizing my
vision for the book. My Creative Director, Andrew Clark, for keeping
my image on track. Paul Cox, an immensely gifted photographer, who
took most of the pictures in this book. David Eldridge, who brought
the design to life. Finally, all the hundreds of talented editors,
photographers, models, stylists, hair and make-up artists with whom
I've had the privilege of working over the years.

Picture Credits

Alpha: pages 51, 57 **Brian Aris**: pages 37, 39, 40 **Nick Briggs**: pages 69, 188

Paul Cox: pages 6, 18, 23, 30, 31, 34, 41, 47, 48, 49, 62, 66, 70, 73, 76, 86, 88, 92, 95, 100, 109, 117, 119, 121, 124, 126, 127, 129, 138, 140, 146, 152, 154, 166, 169, 170, 176, 179, 182, 186, 192, 194, 198, 203, 208, 210, 213, 221, 226, 229, 230

Chris Duffy: pages 5, 68, 104 **Robert Fairer**: pages 113, 115

Fergus Greer: page 158 **Huggy**: page 110 **Stevie Hughes**: page 143 **Trevor Leighton**: page 10

Tony McGee: page 82 **Francois Nars**: page 144 **Terry O'Neill**: pages 27, 107, 156

Iain Philpott: page 32 **Rex Features**: pages 12, 68, 103, 184 **Mario Sorrenti**: page 149

John Swannell: pages 53, 112, 134, 151, 157, 162, 163 **Richard Young**: page 42